Thoracic Surgery in the Elderly

THORACIC SURGERY CLINICS

www.thoracic.theclinics.com

Consulting Editor
MARK K. FERGUSON, MD

August 2009 • Volume 19 • Number 3

SAUNDERS an imprint of ELSEVIER, Inc.

W.B. SAUNDERS COMPANY
A Division of Elsevier Inc.

1600 John F. Kennedy Boulevard • Suite 1800 • Philadelphia, Pennsylvania 19103-2899

http://www.theclinics.com

THORACIC SURGERY CLINICS Volume 19, Number 3
August 2009 ISSN 1547-4127, ISBN-13: 978-1-4377-1391-6, ISBN-10: 1-4377-1391-2

Editor: Catherine Bewick
Developmental Editor: Donald Mumford

Thoracic Surgery Clinics (ISSN 1547-4127) is published quarterly by Elsevier Inc., 360 Park Avenue South, New York, NY 10010-1710. Months of publication are February, May, August, and November. Business and editorial offices: 1600 John F. Kennedy Boulevard, Suite 1800, Philadelphia, PA 19103-2899. Periodicals postage paid at New York, NY, and additional mailing offices. Subscription prices are $242.00 per year (US individuals), $360.00 per year (US institutions), $121.00 per year (US students), $309.00 per year (Canadian individuals), $455.00 per year (Canadian institutions), $165.00 per year (Canadian and foreign students), $329.00 per year (foreign individuals), and $455.00 per year (foreign institutions). Foreign air speed delivery is included in all *Clinics*' subscription prices. All prices are subject to change without notice. **POSTMASTER:** Send address changes to *Thoracic Surgery Clinics*, Elsevier Health Sciences Division, Subscription Customer Service, 3251 Riverport Lane, Maryland Heights, MO 63043. **Customer Service (orders, claims, online, change of address): Telephone: 1-800-654-2452 (U.S. and Canada); 314-447-8871 (outside U.S. and Canada). Fax: 314-447-8029. Email: journalscustomerservice-usa@elsevier.com (for print support); journalsonlinesupport-usa@elsevier.com (for online support).**

Reprints. For copies of 100 or more, of articles in this publication, please contact Commercial Rights Department, Elsevier Inc., 360 Park Avenue South, New York, NY 10010-1710. Tel: (212) 633-3812; Fax: (212) 462-1935; E-mail: reprints@elsevier.com.

Thoracic Surgery Clinics is covered in *MEDLINE/PubMed (Index Medicus)* and *EMBASE/Excerpta Medica*.

Printed and bound by CPI Group (UK) Ltd, Croydon, CR0 4YY

Transferred to Digital Print 2012

Contributors

CONSULTING EDITOR

MARK K. FERGUSON, MD
Professor of Surgery, Section of Cardiac and Thoracic Surgery, The University of Chicago, Chicago, Illinois

AUTHORS

ANITA S. BAGRI, MD
Geriatric Research, Education and Clinical Center, Bruce W. Carter Veterans Affairs Medical Center, Miami, Florida

SARAH BILLMEIER, MD
General Surgery Resident, Brigham and Women's Hospital, Boston, Massachusetts

ILENE BROWNER, MD
Instructor, Department of Oncology and Division of Geriatric Medicine and Gerontology, Johns Hopkins Hospital; Instructor, Department of Medical Oncology, Sidney Kimmel Comprehensive Cancer Center, Johns Hopkins Hospital and Johns Hopkins Bayview Medical Center, Baltimore, Maryland

DEIRDRE M. CAROLAN DOERFLINGER, CRNP, PhD
Geriatrics Clinical Nurse Specialist, Inova Fairfax Hospital, Falls Church, George Mason University, Fairfax, Virginia; George Washington University School of Medicine and Health Sciences, Washington, DC

ANDREW C. CHANG, MD
Assistant Professor of Surgery, Section of General Thoracic Surgery, University of Michigan Health Systems; Comprehensive Cancer Center, University of Michigan Health Systems, Ann Arbor, Michigan

MARIE N. HANNA, MD
Assistant Professor, Department of Anesthesiology and Critical Care Medicine, The Johns Hopkins University, The Johns Hopkins Hospital, Baltimore, Maryland

PAUL M. HEERDT, MD, PhD
Department of Anesthesiology and Pharmacology, Weil Medical College of Cornell University, Critical Care Medicine, Memorial Sloan-Kettering Cancer, New York, New York

HOLLY M. HOLMES, MD
Assistant Professor, Department of General Internal Medicine, Ambulatory Treatment and Emergency Care, The University of Texas M. D. Anderson Cancer Center, Houston, Texas

MICHAEL JAKLITSCH, MD
Associate Professor of Surgery, Director of Clinical Research, Division of Thoracic Surgery, Brigham and Women's Hospital, Boston, Massachusetts

KANUPRIYA KUMAR, MD
Assistant Professor, Department of Anesthesiology and Critical Care Medicine, The Johns Hopkins University, The Johns Hopkins Hospital, Baltimore, Maryland

JULIA S. LEE, MS
Comprehensive Cancer Center, University of Michigan Health Systems, Ann Arbor, Michigan

JOSEPH LoCICERO III, MD
Professor of Surgery, SUNY Downstate; Director of Surgical Oncology, Chief of Thoracic Surgery, Maimonides Medical Center, Brooklyn, New York

M. BLAIR MARSHALL, MD, FACS
Associate Professor of Surgery, Division of Thoracic Surgery, Georgetown University School of Medicine; Chief, Division of Thoracic Surgery, Georgetown University Medical Center, Washington, DC

RITA A. MUKHTAR, MD
Resident, Department of Surgery, University of California, San Francisco, San Francisco, California

JAMIE D. MURPHY, MD
Assistant Professor, Department of Anesthesiology and Critical Care Medicine, The Johns Hopkins University, The Johns Hopkins Hospital, Baltimore, Maryland

BERNARD J. PARK, MD
Department of Surgery, Division of Thoracic Surgery, Memorial Sloan-Kettering Cancer Center, New York, New York

MICHAEL PURTELL, MD, PhD
Assistant Professor, Department of Medical Oncology, Sidney Kimmel Comprehensive Cancer Center, Johns Hopkins Hospital and Johns Hopkins Bayview Medical Center, Baltimore, Maryland

KRISTIN J. REDMOND, MD
Resident Physician, Department of Radiation Oncology and Molecular Radiation Sciences, The Johns Hopkins University School of Medicine, Baltimore, Maryland

ALEX RICO, MD
University of Miami Miller School of Medicine, Miami, Florida

JORGE G. RUIZ, MD
University of Miami Miller School of Medicine; Stein Gerontological Institute, Miami Home and Hospital, Miami, Florida

JASON PHILIP SHAW, MD
Attending Surgeon, Maimonides Medical Center, Brooklyn, New York

DANNY Y. SONG, MD
Assistant Professor, Department of Radiation Oncology and Molecular Radiation Sciences, The Johns Hopkins University School of Medicine, Baltimore, Maryland

PIERRE R. THEODORE, MD
Assistant Professor of Cardiothoracic Surgery, Van Auken Chair in Thoracic Oncology, Department of Surgery, University of California, San Francisco, San Francisco, California

CHRISTOPHER L. WU, MD
Assistant Professor, Department of Anesthesiology and Critical Care Medicine, The Johns Hopkins University, The Johns Hopkins Hospital, Baltimore, Maryland

Contents

Foreword ix

Mark K. Ferguson

Normal Changes of Aging and Their Impact on Care of the Older Surgical Patient 289

Deirdre M. Carolan Doerflinger

Patients 65 years of age or older constitute a large part of the perioperative population. Because the older patient's physiology is unique, it is essential that health care providers recognize the normal physiology of aging and be able to differentiate normal changes of aging from those of pathology. The normal changes of aging result in the older patient presenting differently with specific care needs. Care to this older population must be individualized by providers who are familiar with geriatrics in order to enhance outcomes.

Preoperative Evaluation and Risk Assessment for Elderly Thoracic Surgery Patients 301

Michael Jaklitsch and Sarah Billmeier

The elderly population is growing and increasingly presents for thoracic surgery evaluation. Advancing age has been shown to increase mortality after thoracotomy. Multidisciplinary improvements in perioperative care over the last decades have reduced this risk, making surgical intervention safe for selected patients. A targeted preoperative evaluation helps determine appropriate operative candidates and directs care toward measures to limit or prevent complications. Preoperative assessment in the elderly should include evaluation of cardiopulmonary reserve, comorbidities, and functional and cognitive status. Age alone should not be a contraindication for thoracic surgery.

Benign Thoracic Disease in the Elderly 313

Rita A. Mukhtar and Pierre R. Theodore

Elderly patients present challenges in diagnosis and treatment of various disease processes. Although they may develop thoracic diseases seen in other age groups, older patients often have atypical presentations of these diseases, and may be vulnerable to thoracic pathology as a result of comorbid diseases. Pulmonary function testing of the elderly population shows increased ventilation-perfusion mismatch, decreased forced expiratory volumes, and decreased diffusion capacities. Combined with increased chest wall rigidity, decreasing muscle mass, impaired mucociliary clearance, blunted perception of dyspnea, and possible increased aspiration risk because of underlying neurologic dysfunction, these physiologic changes associated with aging make this population particularly vulnerable to thoracic disease.

Benign Esophageal Disease in the Elderly 321

M. Blair Marshall

The diagnosis and management of benign esophageal disease in the elderly is not necessarily different from that in the general population; however, the comorbidities associated with an aging population are the critical factors that impact morbidity and mortality associated with treatment in this population. Some of the most minimal

Several excellent, non–age-specific review articles and meta-analyses summarize in detail the available trials of surgery and either induction or adjuvant therapy with or without local radiotherapy in the treatment of early non–small cell lung cancer (NSCLC). A detailed review of the literature on the comprehensive assessment of and chemotherapy in the elderly patient with NSCLC is beyond the scope of this article. Instead, the goal is to amalgamate the two topics and develop some practical guidelines to assist the clinician in deciding which therapies most are appropriate for older patients with potentially curable NSCLC.

This article reviews radiation treatment of thoracic malignancies in elderly patients. In general the literature suggests that thoracic irradiation is equally efficacious in elderly patients as in younger patients and is associated with increased but acceptable toxicity. Technical advances are allowing a further reduction in morbidity with preliminary results suggestive of stable outcomes. Prospective data from elderly specific trials are needed to determine the optimal treatment of lung cancer and to compare innovative radiation technology with standard therapies.

With the high burden of lung diseases in the elderly and the rapid aging of the population, thoracic surgeons increasingly will be confronted with the dilemmas that arise in caring for older persons. Providing the optimal treatment for older persons will involve carefully selecting those who have early-stage disease and who are fit for surgery and providing more limited resections to patients who are frailer. Age alone does not determine whether a patient will benefit from thoracic surgery with a reasonable quality of life. Providing appropriate treatment will require a more focused and geriatric-specific evaluation of elderly patients.

Elderly patients (defined as those aged more than 75 years) require specialized care due to the problems associated with deteriorating organ function, minimal organ reserve, blunted responses to stress, and general overall frailty; however, careful, well-planned trials for elderly patients undergoing thoracic surgical procedures have been few, sporadic, and nebulous to date. With the help of the Council on Surgical and Related Medical Specialties of the American Geriatrics Society, a thorough review of the body of literature has been conducted and a research agenda has been defined. Important surgical issues remain to be defined and investigated.

Thoracic Surgery Clinics

FORTHCOMING ISSUES

November 2009

Surgical Conditions of the Diaphragm
Gail Darling, MD, *Guest Editor*

February 2010

Technical Advances in Mediastinal Surgery
Tommaso Claudio Mineo, MD,
Guest Editor

RECENT ISSUES

May 2009

Update on Surgical and Endoscopic Management of Emphysema
Cliff K. Choong, MBBS, FRACS, FRCS,
Guest Editor

February 2009

Diseases of the Mediastinum
Federico Venuta, MD, *Guest Editor*

RELATED INTEREST

Clinics in Geriatric Medicine Volume 24, Issue 4 (November 2008)
Perioperative Management
A.K. Jaffer, MD, *Guest Editor*

Foreword

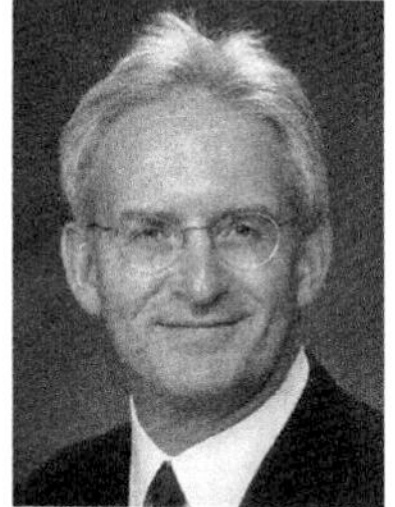

Mark K. Ferguson, MD
Consulting Editor

The elderly population in the United States is growing in size and importance. According to the United States Census Bureau, the United States population that is aged 65 and older grew rapidly for most of the twentieth century, from 3.1 million in 1900 to 35.0 million in 2000. It comprised over 12 percent of the overall population in 2000. Except during the 1990s, the growth of the older population outpaced that of the total population and the population under the age of 65. Despite this apparent slowdown in the growth of the population aged 65 and older during the 1990s, the older population is on the threshold of a boom. According to United States Census Bureau projections, a substantial increase in the number of older people will occur from 2010 to 2030. The older population in 2030 is projected to be twice as large as in 2000, growing from 35 million to 72 million and representing nearly 20 percent of the total United States population at the latter date.

The specialty of thoracic surgery is focused, in a large part, on elderly individuals. The median age for lung cancer resection patients is 65 years, for esophageal cancer patients it is 64 years, and for patients with benign problems such as empyema, the mean age is 56 years. Therefore, among patients upon whom we perform major operations, as many as half can be classified as elderly. This dictates that thoracic surgeons acknowledge the necessity of becoming educated about the special needs of the elderly in our practices. These needs are related not only to alterations in human physiology as the body ages, but are also associated with changes in mood, lifestyle, expectations regarding quality of life, and risk-taking behavior in the elderly population.

This issue of *Thoracic Surgery Clinics* provides a thorough overview of concepts that thoracic surgeons must master when dealing with an ageing population. It begins with articles outlining physiologic changes in the elderly patient and appropriately focuses on the evaluation of older patients for operative risk. In addition, one article specifically targets the evaluation of patients for the risk of postoperative delirium, which is a challenging problem that precipitates physiologic complications and prolongs hospital stay. The subsequent articles outline benign esophageal and pulmonary conditions and their special features in the elderly, and surgical management of lung and esophageal cancer as applied to the older population.

The series of articles on pain management, chemotherapy, and radiation therapy in the ageing population will be of great interest to surgeons. Information regarding these subspecialty management challenges will inform our future discussions with elderly patients about the treatment options that are open to them. One particularly valuable contribution concerns quality of life and outlook in the elderly population. Considerations regarding depression and other mood alterations that accompany the ageing process are very important. In addition, invaluable information is provided about current quality of life and how it affects a patient's decision regarding thoracic surgery, and also how thoracic surgery affects postoperative quality of life. Finally, an article is provided

Thorac Surg Clin 19 (2009) ix–x
doi:10.1016/j.thorsurg.2009.07.006
1547-4127/09/$ – see front matter

that summarizes important shortcomings in our knowledge regarding the elderly patient and outlines methods for bridging this gap through future data collection and research.

Overall, this issue provides important insights into the assessment and the management of the elderly patient who is a candidate for thoracic surgery. As the number of elderly patients grows in the future, there will be an increasing disparity between their number and the number of available geriatricians to help manage the special challenges this population offers. The information provided in this issue of *Thoracic Surgery Clinics* is one small step towards the "geriatricization" of thoracic surgeons. These surgeons will, of necessity, fill the current gap in care of the elderly thoracic surgery patient, enabling geriatricians to focus on the more problematic older patients who truly require subspecialty care.

A number of people were involved in the bringing this issue of *Thoracic Surgery Clinics* to publication, and I'd like to acknowledge the efforts of two individuals in particular. Stephen Yang, MD, was responsible for generating the concept of an issue on thoracic surgery in the elderly, and was instrumental in identifying article content and potential authors. Catherine Bewick, Executive Publisher at Elsevier, has been invaluable in her characteristic proactive, organized way. By keeping the manuscript flow moving despite considerable obstacles, she has facilitated publication of this issue, enabling the reader to enjoy information and recommendations that are authoritative and up to date.

Mark K. Ferguson, MD
Department of Surgery
The University of Chicago Medical Center
5841 S. Maryland Avenue
MC5035
Chicago, IL 60637, USA

E-mail address:
mferguso@surgery.bsd.uchicago.edu

Normal Changes of Aging and Their Impact on Care of the Older Surgical Patient

Deirdre M. Carolan Doerflinger, CRNP, PhD[a,b,c,*]

KEYWORDS

- Changes of aging • Normal aging
- Geriatrics • Elderly • Aged • Skin aging
- Geriatric assessment • Geriatric surgery

CHANGES OF AGING

Aging is a universal and inevitable experience. There is no defined course of aging; rather, it varies with the individual and the variability of aging is increasingly variable the older the patient. The variable rate of decline also increases with advancing age. At birth, initial growth is supplemental. The individual grows, matures, develops, and discovers new abilities. The process of growth continues until adulthood, with some abilities peaking by the age of 30. Other abilities such as learning, judgment, and experience continue to develop over the course of the life span. Alternatively, the changes of aging are considered by some to be detrimental. Although the majority of the population over 65 is functional, independent, healthy, and happy, these changes are commonly viewed as an overall decline.

EPIDEMIOLOGY

The numbers of older individuals in the United States are growing at a rapid rate, with growth projected to continue into the next two decades. In 2004, the most recent year for which data are available, there were 36.3 million individuals 65 years and older in the United States. That group represented 12.4% of the United States population, or one in eight Americans. The number of older Americans has increased 9.3% since 1994. Americans 45 to 64 years old, who will reach 65 in the next 20 years, increased by 39% during the same period. Women over 65 outnumber men at a ratio of 139 to 100. This ratio increases with age; those over 85 have a ratio of 222 to 100. The percentage of Americans 65 years and older tripled from 1900 (4.15%) to 2004 (12.4%). Actual numbers increased from 3.1 million to 36.3 million in 2004.[1]

The older population is projected to get even older owing to better nutrition, better management of chronic disorders, and better health care as a whole. The older population is mushrooming, with the oldest age groups increasing at the most rapid rate. In 2003 persons reaching 65 years of age had an average life expectancy of an additional 18.5 years (19.8 years for females, 16.8 years for males). The group 65 to 74 years old increased eight times since 1900. The group 75 to 84 years old increased 17 times, and those 85 and older increased almost 40 times. Census estimates show an annual net increase of over 375,000 in those 65 years and older. In 2004 there were 64,658 people 100 years and older (0.18% of the total population). This represents a 73% increase from the 1990 number of 37,306.[1]

APPROACH TO THE OLDER PATIENT

The care of the older person—pre-, intra-, and postoperatively—can be positively influenced by

A version of this article originally appeared in the December 2007 issue of Perioperative Nursing Clinics.
[a] Inova Fairfax Hospital, 3300 Gallows Road, Falls Church, VA 22042, USA
[b] George Mason University, Fairfax, VA, USA
[c] George Washington University School of Medicine and Health Sciences, Washington, DC, USA
* Inova Fairfax Hospital, 3300 Gallows Road, Falls Church, VA 22042.
E-mail address: deirdre.carolan@inova.com

Thorac Surg Clin 19 (2009) 289–299
doi:10.1016/j.thorsurg.2009.06.007

a number of factors. A positive, unbiased attitude, interdisciplinary collaboration, and incorporation into care of validated assessment tools increase accuracy of assessments and promote improved outcomes. The examiner must evaluate his or her own attitudes toward the older patient to increase awareness of personal bias and prevent stereotyping of the elderly.[2,3]

Communication must be enhanced in order to be clear to the patient, the patient's family or home caregivers, and the medical physician managing care. It is paramount to excellent outcomes that communication among the care team be as clear and concise as possible.[4] Premorbid functional assessment, preferably using standardized assessment tools such as the Katz Activities of Daily Living Index or Lawton and Brody's Instrumental Activities of Daily Living, should be conducted to weigh the risk/benefit ratio with the patient and his or her family.[2,5–8] (Both tools and many others are available free of charge at http://www.geronurseonline.org/.)

Additionally, assessment and identification of depression in older individuals increase the effectiveness of treatment and avert hazards to recovery.[9] The use of the Geriatric Depression Scale is more accurate in the older population than are nonspecific tools.[5] Multiple, well-managed medical conditions such as hypertension, glaucoma, peripheral neuropathy, and osteoporosis may be less of a consideration and less limiting than a single diagnosis of advanced dementia.

Psychosocial assessment should include ethnic factors, cultural considerations, and the social supports that are currently in place.[5,9–13] Poorly managed or uncontrolled comorbidities, frailty, and lack of social supports are the significant threats to achieving excellent outcomes in the older surgical patient. The most potentially dangerous error, however, is the assumption that presenting or developing problems are normal changes of aging. It is essential that the health care team be able to distinguish between normal changes of aging with its incumbent impact and those of pathology.[4,6,14–17]

Diagnostic Considerations

Complicating the care of the elder patient is the atypical presentation of illness in many older adults. The physical changes of aging and accompanying comorbidities require new knowledge and set of skills.[6,7,10,11,14,15] At the age of 85, a person's multiple comorbididities, polypharmacy, and cognitive or functional impairment are predictors of nonspecific presentations. Failure to recognize the atypical presentations of different illnesses of older adults results in increased morbidity and mortality, missed diagnoses, and unnecessary emergency visits and hospitalizations. Atypical presentations generally fall into three categories: vague illness, altered presentation of illness, and nonpresentation or underreporting of illness.[4,7,11,14,15]

Vague presentations of illness

Common vague presentations of illness that may be seen are confusion, self-neglect, new or increasing falls, urinary incontinence, anorexia or weight loss, and fatigue. Any changes in behavior or function in older adults, especially in the very frail, can indicate an acute disease or a developing condition. Subtle signs must be given serious consideration by the health care team. Careful attention to family and caregiver observations is warranted.[10,11,14,15,18]

Altered presentation of illness

Older patients may also present with altered presentation of an illness. Classic presentations seen in a younger population cannot be generalized to the older patient. Depression, acute abdomen, malignancy, pulmonary edema, myocardial infarction, thyroid disease—all may present uncharacteristically in the older patient.[11,19,20]

Depression Depression prevalence in older adults is estimated from 5% to 40%.[9] Examiners may view the older depressed patients as having justified reasons for sadness and fail to treat them. Depressed older patients may present in an agitated or anxious state, many times with intermittent confusion and inability to concentrate. Initial presentation may be frequent visits for vague somatic complaints such as abdominal discomfort, or other intestinal symptoms, constipation, or sleep disturbances. An underlying medical disorder may actually be the presenting issue. Multiple medical problems with their resultant symptoms complicate the diagnosis of depression.[4,11,13]

Thyroid disease Agitation, confusion, and altered cognition are not uncommon presentations of older patients with hypothyroid. Apathetic hyperthyroid condition, a more common disorder in the older patient, presents with fatigue and psychomotor slowing. Vague presenting symptoms resemble a traditional concept of depression and are commonly overlooked. Both disorders may be mistaken as early dementia by clinicians inexperienced in geriatrics, again further delaying treatment.[11,18,19,21–23]

Infections Older adults may not display textbook signs and symptoms of infection. Their presentation may be without leukocytosis, and normal or low-grade fever. Anorexia and decline in function may be the initial signs of sepsis. The most common sources of infection are the respiratory system, urinary system, and the skin or gastrointestinal tract. Cognitively impaired patients should be assessed for infection with an increase in falls, change in mental status, or change in function.[7,10,11,14,24–27]

Myocardial infarction The most common presentation of myocardial infarction in the older patient is an atypical picture; chest pain is rarely present. Dyspnea, an earlier and more classic symptom, is seen far more commonly. Identification of those individuals at risk is essential for earlier recognition of the vague symptoms of nausea, change in mental status, fatigue, and functional decline that are more frequently seen in this population.[6,7,14,28]

Pulmonary edema The classic symptoms of increased fluid retention, dyspnea, and fatigue associated with congestive heart failure are commonly seen in the elderly. Persistent cough may not be recognized as a symptom by the older patient. Again, sole presentation may develop subtly, and with only the vague symptoms of nausea, change in mental status, fatigue, and functional decline.[7,24,28,29]

Acute abdomen The older adult with an acute abdominal process may present silently. Sole complaints may be abdominal discomfort, nausea, and fatigue. Respiratory complaints are seen with higher frequency than in a younger population. The caregiver should carefully monitor for bowel distress; decreased oral intake should be encouraged.[7,11,14,30,31]

Malignancy Age is the major risk for malignancy. Compliance with preventative screenings may be hampered by mobility, access, and lack of awareness of the impact of cancer. Although many cancers may follow an indolent course in the older patient, significant impact is felt from later diagnosis. Back pain or surface breast lesions may be the presenting symptoms leading to diagnosis of metastatic disease. Irregular bowel function may be ignored or accepted as a normal change of aging, thus delaying diagnosis of intestinal malignancy.[6,7,11,14,17,30–32]

Absent presentation of illness

Many disorders in the elderly that are not identified or treated routinely have major implications for quality of life. Cognitive dysfunction such as depression and dementia increase lack of recognition of the sensory deficits of hearing loss, visual deterioration, and declining dental health. Mobility issues such as osteoporosis, arthritis, and reduced flexibility may elude recognition and therefore treatment. Quality of life deteriorates if falls, poor nutrition, or incontinence is not recognized and addressed. A host of illnesses in older adults may go unrecognized for many years and significantly impact quality of life.[7,12,14,17]

Issues compromising the recognition of disease are, in some cases, the gradual onset and vague symptomatology with which they present. Many symptoms of disease are seen as normal changes of aging by caregivers. Stoicism of the older adult and misperception of normal aging by the patient are impediments to reporting developing symptoms, as is the worry of testing and fear of bad news. Fears of possible loss of independence, expense, and physical discomfort are all concerns expressed by older adults. Reporting may also be hampered by cognitive impairment, inability to verbalize symptoms, and concerns that the elderly will not be taken seriously.[2–4,6,11,14,24,28,29,31,33]

Changes of Aging

The process of aging affects every cell, tissue, organ, and organism. Most systems have specific changes, whereas a few systems have vague deregulatory changes. Changes are due to a combination of factors, genetics, environment, nutrition, and activity, all of which are influential. Changes of aging are not harmful in isolation, but physiologic resilience is compromised. Homeostasis becomes more difficult to maintain when stressed.[4,12,17,19,20,24,26]

Cardiovascular system

In the older population, the heart itself will have increased weight. Left ventricular hypertrophy is a frequent finding. Decreased force of contraction is commonly present, as is valvular sclerosis. There is a decline in the number of pacer cells, and those remaining demonstrate reduced efficiency. There is a reduced beta adrenergic response. Decreased vascular compliance, arterial wall stiffening, and wall thickening are frequently seen. A dilated aorta is a common finding, and tissues can have reduced oxygen uptake.[4,12,17,19,20,24,26]

Changes due to aging in the cardiovascular system result in decreased cardiac reserve and decreased cardiac output. A decline in maximum heart rate is seen, with heart rates ranging from 40 to 100 beats per minute. The older patient recovers more slowly from tachycardia and commonly experiences fatigue and shortness of breath. Changes in the pacing cells may be seen in increased numbers of premature or ectopic beats. Extra heart sounds are common, with the S4 heard most often. A finding of an S3 is always abnormal.[7] There is increased risk of valvular dysfunction in the older patient and increased risk of systolic murmurs. The older patient regularly exhibits a systolic ejection murmur at the left lower sternal border with no pathologic compromise.[10,18,19,26–28] There is higher risk of conduction abnormalities, postural- and diuretic-induced hypotension, and higher risk of carotid artery buckling and jugular venous distention. Inflamed varicosities are more common. Systolic blood pressure is frequently increased, and is accompanied by increases in pulse pressure and peripheral resistance. Strong arterial pulses are present; diminished peripheral pulses and cool extremities are regularly seen.[4,12,18,20,24,26,27]

Implications Blood pressure should be assessed with the patient lying, sitting, and standing. Pulse pressures should be assessed at the same time. Auscultate the heart for murmurs, rubs, or gallops and note heart rate and rhythm. Document any abnormal findings such as altered landmarks, distant heart sounds, or displaced point of maximal impact. Carotid arteries, internal jugulars, and varicosities should be assessed. Check the ECG for arrhythmias and other changes. Incorporate into the assessment the patient's function and mobility.[5,10,11]

Referral should be considered for those patients with new or rapid arrhythmias, irregularities in heart function, or altered blood flow. Validation of patient understanding of orthostatic hypotension should be confirmed, as should the patient's and family's knowledge of the recommended safety precautions for patients with orthostatic hypotension. These precautions should include rising slowly from lying or sitting or delaying further position change for 1 to 2 minutes. Monitor the patient and ensure that his or her family recognizes overt signs of hypotension such as sensorial or mental status changes or dizziness. Patients exhibiting compromise on their cardiac exam should be assessed for risk of falling; institute fall prevention strategies.[3–6,12,15,20]

Respiratory system

The examiner will find increased rigidity of the thorax and vertebrae. Older patients also display decreased muscle strength and reduced endurance. The older lung has diminished ciliary activity and decreased macrophage activity in addition to increased airway reactivity. Mucous membranes are drier. The lungs will have decreased alveolar function and reduced vascularization and elastic recoil. Decreased response to hypoxia and hypercarbia will be seen.[4,5,12,19,20,24,26,29]

The older patient may present with kyphosis and a barrel-shaped rigid chest. Respiratory rate should remain stable at 12 to 24 respirations per minute. Examiners may note decreased respiratory excursion and reduced chest expansion with compromised exhalation. Diminished breath sounds, especially in lung bases, are frequently noted. Risk of infection and asthma are increased owing to decreased cough and compromised deep breathing with subsequent impaired clearance of foreign matter. Altered pulmonary function may present as lower maximal expiratory flow, increased residual volume, or reduced vital capacity in the presence of unchanged total lung capacity. The patient presents commonly with dyspnea after exertion and decreased exercise tolerance. Decreased partial pressure of oxygen and saturation of peripheral oxygen are present in addition to compromise in maintenance of acid/base balance.[4,12,19,20,24,26,29]

Implications Assess respirations and breath sounds in all lung fields. Thorax appearance and chest expansion should be checked. Assess cough, deep breathing, and exercise capacity. Assess the older patient for asthma, chronic obstructive pulmonary disease, and other conditions that may compromise respiratory function. Monitor the individual for early signs of pulmonary infections. If clinically indicated, monitor oxygenation using arterial blood gases and pulse oximetry.[5] Check for secretions, sedation, or positioning that might impair oxygenation or ventilation. Positioning, suctioning, and excellent pulmonary toilet should be used to maintain patient airway and avert pulmonary infection. The patient and family should be instructed in use of incentive spirometry. If there is an inability to ambulate or a new decline in function, education on coughing, avoidance of environmental hazards, and smoking cessation should be included.[2,4–6,10,12,16,20,29,34–36]

Genitourinary system

The genitourinary system has multiple components. The renal changes of aging have more impact on the health and care of the older patient, but the aging bladder may have more social and functional implications. The kidney is responsible for the maintenance of baseline homeostasis for fluid/electrolyte balances. Glomeruli die and are not replaced. Minimal stress on the renal system may not present a problem; however, the stress of disease or trauma may present an impact. The older kidney has decreased functional reserve when there is an imbalance in water or sodium both in overload or deficit conditions. The older kidney weighs less than its younger counterpart and has less blood flow, decreased oxygenation, and a reduced glomerular filtration rate, frequently of less than 50%. These changes increase the importance of creatinine clearance measurement or use of an estimated creatinine clearance formula before the older patient is medicated. There is tubular degeneration seen corresponding with a lower glomerular filtration rate. The aging kidney responds less efficiently to vasopressin and has impaired capacity to dilute, concentrate, and acidify urine. Impaired sodium regulation issues may present at this time.[18,20,24,27]

The bladder becomes less elastic with reduced muscle tone and a smaller capacity with age. Detrusor instability, involuntary bladder contractions, and a weakened urinary sphincter may threaten continence. Many older individuals experience decreased or delayed perception of voiding signals. When accompanied by increased nocturnal production of urine, this can lead to interrupted sleep or self-imposed fluid restriction. Normal human prostatic fluid possesses pronounced antibacterial activity.[37] As men age, they are at risk of decreased prostatic antibacterial factor and benign prostatic hyperplasia.[36] Older postmenopausal females experience estrogen loss, decreased pelvic area elasticity, and atrophy of gland and epithelial tissue. Concurrently, the vaginal pH becomes more alkaline.[18,20,24,27]

Changes related to aging in the genitourinary system increase both the risk of renal complications in illness and the susceptibility to acute ischemic renal failure and embolism. The risk of dehydration is increased, as is the vulnerability to volume overload. Hyperkalemia related to potassium-sparing diuretics is seen, as is hyponatremia associated with thiazide diuretics. Hypernatremia is seen with use of nonsteroidal anti-inflammatory drugs.

The older patient will have reduced excretion of their acid load via the renal system and increased risk of postural hypotension. Decreased drug clearance must be a consideration when treating this population. Careful selection of drugs and dosage modification is essential. There is increased risk of nephrotoxic injury by pharmacologic agents.[18,20,24,27]

In spite of the changes in the genitourinary system, the older person will have normal renal function and constant serum creatinine level and should be absent proteinuria. Increased postvoid residual may be noted, placing the individual at increased risk of urinary tract infection and incontinence, neither of which are normal findings. Nocturia and polyuria are both risk factors for falls. The older male is at risk of urinary hesitancy, dribbling, frequency, and incontinence. The older female is at risk for atrophic vaginitis, urethritis, vaginal stenosis, and vaginal or uterine prolapse.[18,20,24,27,35,36]

Implications Renal function should be assessed, especially in the presence of acute or chronic illness. Estimates of renal function should be obtained using the Cockcroft Gault equation. For men, the calculation is creatinine clearance (mL/min) = 140-age (years) × body weight (kg) divided by 72 × serum creatinine (mg/dL). For women, multiply this number by 0.85 because of lower muscle mass in the female body.[4,8,11,16,20,35,36] Monitor blood pressure on all older patients to enhance early identification and intervention of orthostasis. Assess these patients for dehydration, volume overload, electrolyte imbalances, and proteinuria. Identify the etiology of fluid and electrolyte imbalance. Monitor labs reflecting renal function for changes. Palpate the bladder after voiding to determine whether retention is an issue and assess for urinary incontinence. In men, assess urine stream for abnormalities common with benign prostatic hyperplasia. Place the patient on falls precautions if urgency, nocturia, or frequency is present.[17,20,24,37] Teach the patient and family coping strategies for postural hypotension, such as slow position changes with rest periods between movements. Nephrotoxic drugs and renally excreted medications should be selected carefully, and the risk and benefit of the medication should be considered. If problems are impeding function, consider referral to incontinence, renal, or urology specialists as needed.[6,8,11,12,16,18,20,24,26]

Integumentary system

The major skin concerns in the surgical arena are twofold. Skin is essential in maintaining body temperature, and older skin heals more slowly. Consideration needs to be given to the maintenance of skin integrity in any prolonged surgery or where hypotensive episodes are routine. Changes reflecting skin aging are the result of three factors: sun damage, chronologic aging, and hormonal influences. The majority of aging changes are a consequence of cumulative sun exposure.[3,10–12,33] Chronologic aging represents those changes that occur in nonexposed areas of the body. The changes that occur in the integumentary system are a result of decreased subcutaneous fat, decreased interstitial fluid, decreased muscle tone, decreased glandular activity, and reduced efficiency of sensory receptors. Collagen stiffens, there is reduced blood supply, and the ability to repair declines with age. There is increased capillary fragility.[6,10,11,20,33] Hair is affected by changes of aging in that there is a thinning and graying of hair and decreased melanin production. Blood supply slows to the fingernails. These changes result in cool, pale, dry skin in the older adult. Increased fragility, wrinkling, tenting, and sagging of skin occur and increase the risk of yeast infections.[12,20,27,33] The ability to maintain temperature is affected predominantly by decreased perspiration coupled with the loss of subcutaneous fat.[20,25] This is accompanied by decreased elasticity, turgor, increased risk of skin tears, ecchymosis, dermatitis, pressure ulcers, and dehydration. The older patient will have increased lentigines and neoplasm. Sensation is decreased with the consequential increased risk of injury. Fat is decreased throughout the body, and loss of fat, in addition to deterioration of muscle tone, can affect ambulation. Nails become thick and brittle and split easily, increasing risk of fungal infections.[10,20,27,33,38]

Implications Skin should be monitored for changes in temperature, turgor, hydration status, changes in color, pigmentation, lesions, and bruising. Intertriginous areas (areas of skin folding) should be cleaned, dried, and regularly assessed for fungal infections. Monitor feet for the need for podiatry interventions. Older patients should be assessed regularly for risk of skin breakdown and appropriate interventions implemented. Patients and families may be following usual norms of daily hot showers that may not be indicated for aging skin. New or changing lesions on the skin should be assessed for the potential for malignancy and referred to dermatology in a timely fashion. In the operating room, care must be taken to monitor the environment and the patient to maintain body temperature and prevent hypothermia or hyperthermia. Adequate fluids—preferably oral, but if not, then intravenous—should be maintained to prevent dehydration.[16,17,25,30,32,38,39]

Gastrointestinal system

The older patient will commonly have decreased thirst perception, decreased saliva, and dry mucosa. There may be bone loss in the jaw and bone surrounding teeth. There are atrophy and loss of taste buds and atrophy of olfactory receptors.[20,40] The older patient will exhibit decreased esophageal motility and decreases in lower esophageal sphincter pressure. Decreased motility extends through the stomach, accompanied by mucosal atrophy, and the small and large intestines. There are reduced and less efficient small intestinal villi and digestive enzyme secretion. The slowing in the large intestine is compounded by decreased blood flow and defecation sensation. The liver experiences decreased size, decreased blood flow, and decreased enzymatic metabolism of drugs. The pancreas has decreased reserve and decreased enzymatic and hormonal secretory cells.[4,10,12,18–20,24,26,27]

The changes in the digestive system may result in impaired digestive ability and increases in food intolerances. The risk of dehydration is magnified, as is the risk of electrolyte imbalances. Nutritional intake may be inadequate owing to multiple factors of loneliness and inability to access and prepare food. Impaired sense of smell and taste (many times exacerbated by medications) and the loss of taste of foods once enjoyed are also contributing factors.[4,6,12,18,20,26,41,42] There is increased incidence of gingivitis, and these older patients may present with significant tooth loss. Altered muscle tone in the gastrointestinal tract and delayed gastric emptying further predispose the older patient to increased risk of dysphagia, hiatal hernia, aspiration, and gastroesophageal reflux disease.[6,31] The older person may have inefficient absorption of fat, carbohydrates, proteins, B_{12}, iron, folate, vitamin D, and calcium. These deficiencies contribute to increased risk of malnutrition, osteoporosis, and anemia. Common complaints from the older patient are constipation and flatulence.[31] With slowed motility, the risk of fecal impaction increases. An increase in the incidence of cholecystolithiasis has been observed.[31]

Implications Weight change, especially loss, is a significant indicator of well-being in the older patient and should be monitored with each interaction. The abdomen should be assessed in the routine fashion, as should the oral cavity for dentition, chewing, and swallowing. Smaller liver size will be percussed. Dietary intake and elimination patterns should be elicited and noted. If the patient is deemed at risk for aspiration, a careful pulmonary exam is warranted. Education on nutrition and diet has the potential to increase the older person's nutritional status. Simple instructions, including fluid intake, toileting, and bowel health, can significantly lessen the impact of these changes on the person's quality of life.[10,20,24]

Musculoskeletal system

Routinely, the older patient has narrowed intervertebral disks, decreased cortical and trabecular bone mass, and replacement of lean body mass by adipose tissue. Muscle fiber mass is diminished, and muscle fibers are not replaced as efficiently. Muscle contraction time is increased. There is increased flexion of the hip and knee and ligament stiffening. Joints are affected to varying degrees by calcium deposits, cartilage erosion, and bony overgrowth and spurs.[3,6,17,20,26,43] The musculoskeletal system exhibits increasing variability in age-related changes among individuals, and this diversity is exaggerated by increasing age. Kyphosis may cause height loss, which may be minimal or significant. Balance and therefore gait and stability are commonly affected. There is increased incidence of osteoarthritis and osteoporosis and increased risk and numbers of fractures. Fat, in the body, shifts from extremities to become more centrally stored. There is less total body water and fluid, in both intercellular and interstitial storage. This further increases risk of fluid and electrolyte imbalances. Muscle agility is decreased, as is muscle strength. Reaction times become prolonged, and the patient may have slowed deep tendon reflexes. Overall, the older patient may exhibit decreased exercise endurance and mobility and is at increased risk of musculoskeletal injury.[3,4,20,24,27,43]

Implications The most essential element of assessment in the older patient is functionality. This assessment should include mobility, fine motor and gross motor skills, and activities of daily living. Examination should be carefully performed to ensure joint stability. Slow, gentle, passive movements should be used to assess range of motion. The patient should be encouraged to follow a regular exercise program, the components of which should be discussed. Maximal benefit will occur by including aerobic exercise in addition to muscle strengthening and balance. The older patient garners significant benefit from physical or occupational therapy consultation and information on environmental modifications to maximize function.[4,20,24,27,43]

Nervous system

Nervous system changes related to aging are viewed as loss of function and abilities. The adult brain, however, continues to have the ability to compensate for those losses that occur. Wisdom, experience, and perception remain stable or improve with age. The size and weight of the brain decrease owing to atrophy, which predominantly affects the gray matter. Older nerve cells have fewer dendrites and they are more likely to be demyelinated, slowing neural transmission. Most changes in the nervous system occur after age 60. There is a higher incidence of cognitive impairment in the older adult, with a third of those over the age of 85 suffering from some cognitive changes. As with function, cognitive abilities vary with the individual.[4,6,10–12,18,20,34,39]

Specific spheres of cognitive function are affected differently by changes of aging. Learning time is commonly extended in those older than 70. Reaction times are slower and short-term memory is slightly decreased. Attention is maintained or improved with age. Language skills overall are not affected, although word retrieval does decrease. Objective assessment of memory demonstrates minimal changes.[18–20] Older adults performed less well on encoding, retention, and retrieval testing. Memory changes, overall, in the healthy brain are minimal. At all ages recall is worse than recognition. Recall declines with age while recognition is preserved intact. Long-term memory remains relatively stable. Visuospatial ability declines, as does abstraction. Problem solving tends to decline with age, whereas verbal scores remain stable. If declines occur, it is usually after age 70. Declining with age are mental flexibility and abstract thinking, especially among those 70 and older.[18–20]

Implications The older patient may experience declining reflexes and decreased or slowed processing. The ability to interpret multiple stimuli is slowed.[10,24,40] Multiple simultaneous tasks become more difficult to manage. The older individual may exhibit gait disturbance, which may have a musculoskeletal basis but frequently is a result of altered or impaired proprioception. Gait abnormalities, coupled with poor balance, increased incidence of parasthesias, and the potential for hypotension, increase the risk of falls. Pain sensation threshold is increased.[30,32,39] This population will present with wide variation in cognitive function. All older patients should be screened for early cognitive impairment in order to enhance quality of life and care planning. Monitor this individual for orthostasis. Consider a home evaluation for modification of the environment. Assess caregiver needs and concerns and address them. Patient teaching will need to be modified to allow increased time for information to be presented and encoded by the older patient.[4,17–20,26,38]

The senses

Touch The sense of touch in the older patient is diminished owing to an overall decline in the number of touch receptors in all parts of the body. Patient response to pain is decreased. Touch predominantly affects personal safety: lack of sensation of extreme heat, coupled with delayed reflexes, results in a higher number of burns in the home. These burns tend to be worse than those of a younger patient.[10,18,20,34,40]

Awareness of the decrease in touch receptors, along with an elevated pain threshold, significantly increases risk for burns and other injuries. Careful precautions should be taken with positioning any external devices or fluids not at room temperature.[38,40]

Taste The older person frequently complains of food not tasting good, tasting as in the past, or tasting differently. There are a number of mechanisms contributing to this effect. Receptor cells are found in the taste buds on the tongue. In youth, these are constantly dying and being replaced. With age, actual number of taste buds diminishes and the tongue and remaining taste buds atrophy. Loss of teeth from decay may lead to atrophy of the jaw, absent dentures or poorly fitting appliances.[4,20,27,31,40]

Regular monitoring of weight is the most effective mechanism to ensure adequate intake. Use of seasoning to enhance flavor, in addition to allowing food preferences, may increase intake. Dietary assessment and interventions may also be helpful in maintaining adequate nutrition. If issues with nutrition persist, the patient's feelings regarding artificial feeding should be assessed.[31,40,42,44,45]

Smell With age there is a decrease in the number of smell receptors, and those remaining function less efficiently. This increases the threshold for smell. For the older person to identify a smell, it must be more intense and markedly different from surrounding scents. Smell decreases rapidly after a person reaches 50 years of age. The sense of smell has declined by 50% by the 80s.[18,20,26,27,31,40]

The sense of smell is a protective mechanism. Detection of spoiled food prior to eating is impaired. Older individuals may not be aware of warning smells such as smoke, burning, or gas leaks until there is a serious emergency or explosion.[12,31,40]

Visual and hearing impairment Among older individuals, 75% have significant impairment in their hearing and/or vision. These impairments may go unreported by the patient and unrecognized by family and health care providers. These impairments frequently result in social isolation, decreased function, and decreased communication. The individual may appear cognitively impaired.[18–20,40]

Vision The eye may be one of the earliest systems to display changes related to normal aging. Many of the changes are more subtle than visual acuity. Orbital fat decreases with age, as does muscle elasticity and tear production. There is decreased corneal sensitivity and reflex. Loss of pigment in the iris may be seen; the pupil may decrease in size. Within the eye there is increased vitreous gel debris and decreased aqueous humor secretion, with reduced cleansing of the lens and the cornea.[18,19,26,40] Ciliary muscles atrophy and the lens becomes yellowed, denser, and less elastic. Less light is conducted to the retina. The older eye may become dry and recede. Upward gaze may become limited. On exam, extraocular movements remain intact. Arcus senilis, which may be seen commonly as a gray halo around the cornea, is formed by lipid deposition at the periphery of the cornea but has no clinical significance. There is increased risk of ectropion, entropion, conjunctivitis, infection, senile ptosis, and corneal abrasion owing to decreased sensation of the cornea and changes in the structure of the orbit. The older patient may report blurred vision and decreased visual acuity—more pronounced in low light and in the presence of glare.[8,12,18,19,26,27,40] Vitreous floaters are a more common complaint in the older adult. Aging causes presbyopia, decreased peripheral vision, impaired light accommodation, decreased color discrimination, impaired night vision, and impaired depth perception. The older adult needs more light to see clearly and easily. The older, smaller pupil complicates the examination of the retina. Risks of injury, cataracts, and narrow-angle glaucoma increase with age.[10,12,18,20,24,27,40]

Visual acuity should be assessed under different lighting, and color discrimination should be assessed more frequently. Visual limitations have the potential to limit driving, ambulation, and safety in general. In the social setting, visual changes impact social interactions and safety in the home. A home safety inspection can facilitate remediation with lighting and elimination of hazards. The older individual should be educated on the importance of regular eye exams to preserve vision. He or she should also be provided information about positive lighting changes to enhance function and about newly developing driving hazards and techniques to prevent falls.[18,19,26,34,40]

Auditory system The changes related to normal aging in the ear are both structural and functional. The aging ear develops ossicular joint deterioration; tympanic membrane thins and is less resilient. Inner ear changes include atrophy of vestibular structures, cochlea, and organ of Corti. The canal contains fewer ceruminal glands, and cerumen produced is drier and harder, with increased risk of impactions and accompanying loss of hearing. Decreased sound conduction and hearing loss are commonly experienced.

High-pitched tones are usually lost earlier. Risk of hearing loss and tinnitus increases, equilibrium declines, and balance deficits are commonly seen.[12,18–20,40]

During examination, the older patient's ear should be assessed for wax buildup and impaction, which can be removed by irrigation and curette. Ensure that any hearing aides are functional, with working batteries and correct placement. If impairment is noted and the patient has not had an audiologic examination, one should be encouraged. Face the older patient when speaking, and make sure there is not background glare obscuring his or her view. Speak slowly in a low pitch voice; avoid raising the voice or yelling. Eliminate as much background noise as possible. Monitor balance and equilibrium and assess risk for falls. Arrange to have the home environment assessed and educate the patient and caregiver on modifications to enhance safety.[8,10,11,34,40]

Hearing impairment has the potential to isolate an older individual. If the patient cannot benefit from or use a hearing aide, use a portable amplifier with headphones if available. (A Pocket Talker is one example of a device that enhances social interactions and improves independence and function.) If temporary assistive technology is not available, a stethoscope can serve the same purpose. Place the earpieces in the patient's ears and speak quietly into the diaphragm. Allow the older person adequate time to process and respond to interactions. These individuals are hearing impaired, not cognitively impaired. Speak to the hearing-impaired patient with the same respect as would be extended to a nonimpaired individual.[18–20,40]

Endocrine

Changes of normal aging affecting the endocrine system have an impact in multiple areas affecting health and function. The systems most affected are the skeletal system, the hormonal system, and fluid and electrolyte homeostasis. Mineral metabolism is impaired owing to reduced efficiency of vitamin D synthesis, estrogen decline, and reduced parathyroid hormone.[18,19,23,24,26] Carbohydrate metabolism is affected by decreased insulin secretion and increased insulin resistance. Decreased renin-angiotensin-aldosterone activity may affect fluid and electrolyte balance, and the older person's ability to maintain homeostasis may be compromised. Body composition is affected by reduced growth hormone and altered glucocorticoid and testosterone activity. The older individual has decreased adrenal functional reserve and a less effective hormonal response.[11,18–20,24]

Overall, basal carbohydrate metabolism remains intact, but challenge will result in decreased glucose tolerance and there is increased risk of type 2 diabetes.[18,19,23,44] Changes in bone metabolism accelerate bone mineral density loss and increase the risk of osteoporosis and fractures. There is increased risk of fluid and electrolyte imbalances and postural hypotension. Body composition changes as fat increases, muscle and bone mass decreases, and strength and functionality may decline, thereby increasing the risk of falls. The fall that occurs has increased risk of injury. Also seen is significant risk of compromised functionality owing to declining response to physiologic stressors triggered by adrenal changes.[10,23,27,43,44]

Implications Thorough assessment of functionality, including risk of falls, fluid and nutritional intake, elimination, and orthostatic blood pressures, is paramount. Fasting and postprandial blood sugar levels as well as bone mineral density should be monitored and reassessed at regular office visits.

The patient should be educated on the importance of nutrition in maintaining health and promoting postoperative healing. Clear guidelines for adequate fluid intake should be emphasized.[8,15,23,42]

Other considerations

The older patient's independence is commonly at risk in today's health care system because of misunderstandings regarding decision-making ability. Cognitive impairment of any kind is considered as an automatic loss of autonomy and the right to self-determination. Competency is the issue raised with the cognitively impaired older adult. The real issue is capacity.

There are usually areas in which the individual can still fully understand the issues, options, and consequences of an action or situation and remain able to make his or her own decisions. Cognitive disorders occur along a continuum of severity—from minimal, which may be unnoticed in the majority of interactions and range in the patient, to extremely severe, which presents with complete disorientation or vegetative symptoms. Careful assessment of the patient's executive function clarifies the areas in which he or she is capable of making decisions, and attempts should be made to allow as much control as is safe. A particular patient may not be able to balance a checkbook and manage finances, but that individual could still be able to designate a surrogate decision maker.[9–11,18,20]

SUMMARY

All health care professionals will at some point come into contact with elderly patients. The older population is increasing in numbers never seen before. Older patients present uniquely in the health care setting. Their bodies have specific changes as a result of aging that impact all facets of their health care. Pain, debility, loss of function, and many other symptoms are expected by the older person and their family and accepted as a fact associated with aging.

Every system in the human body undergoes changes related to aging. Recognition of normal changes of aging will allow the health care provider to identify atypical presentations of illness owing to changes in aging, allowing earlier and more effective treatment. It is incumbent upon all nurses to learn to differentiate normal changes of aging from pathology and to use evidence-based geriatrics practices to improve care of seniors.

ACKNOWLEDGMENTS

The author thanks Anna Herbst, RN, MSN, and Lorraine Taylor, RN, MSN, for their assistance in reviewing this article.

REFERENCES

1. US Bureau of Census. U.S. Bureau of the Census and the National Center for Health Statistics. Available at: http://www.aoa.gov/PROF/Statistics/profile/2005/3.asp. Accessed March 17, 2007.
2. Long M. Attitudinal issues, myths and stereotypes of aging. In: Luggen A, Meiner S, editors. NGNA core curriculum for gerontological nursing. 2nd edition. Philadelphia: Mosby Publishing; 2001. p. 9–14.
3. Mamaril ME. Nursing considerations in the geriatric surgical patient: the perioperative continuum of care. Nurs Clin North Am 2006;41:313–28.
4. Ham R, Sloane D, Warshaw G. Primary care geriatrics: a case based approach. p. 20–8.
5. Meiner S. Assessment of older adults. In: Luggen A, Meiner S, editors. NGNA core curriculum for gerontological nursing. 2nd edition. Philadelphia: Mosby Publishing; 2001. p. 46–52.
6. Kane R, Ouslander J, Abrass I, editors. Essentials of clinical geriatrics. 5th edition. New York: McGraw Hill Publishing; 2004. p. 3–7, 10–4, 35–44, 46–8, 93–110, 295, 296, 480, 490.
7. Flaherty E, Zwicker D. Atypical presentations in the elderly. Available at: http://www.geronurseonline.org/index.cfm?section_id=36&;geriatric_topic_id=16&sub_section_id=101&page_id=234&tab=2. Accessed March 10, 2007.
8. Furstenberg A. Rules for aging: how to manage growing older. principles for responding to age-related changes. J Gerontol Soc Work 1994;23:223–44. Available at: http://www.cinahl.com/cgi-bin/refsvc?jid=826&;accno=1995022055.
9. Brautigan R, Reno B. Psychiatric and psychological problems. In: Luggen A, Meiner S, editors. NGNA core curriculum for gerontological nursing. 2nd edition. Philadelphia: Mosby Publishing; 2001. p. 143–8.
10. Batchelor N. Normal aging changes. In: Luggen A, Meiner S, editors. NGNA core curriculum for gerontological nursing. 2nd edition. Philadelphia: Mosby Publishing; 2001. p. 4–9.
11. Cassel CK, editor. Geriatric medicine: an evidence-based approach. 4th edition. New York: Springer Publishing; 2003. p. 17, 18, 21–3, 26–34, 149, 242–53, 361–6, 695–706, 869–79, 1163–8.
12. Kain CD, Reilly N, Schultz ED. The older adult: a comparative assessment. Nurs Clin North Am 1990;25:833–48. Available at: http://www.cinahl.com/cgi-bin/refsvc?jid=261&;accno=1991117722.
13. Sadavoy J, editor. Comprehensive textbook of geriatric psychiatry. 3rd edition. New York: W.W. Norton; 2004.
14. Amella EJ. Presentation of illness in older adults. If you think you know what you're looking for, think again. AORN J 2006;83:372–4.
15. Amella EJ. Presentation of illness in older adults. Am J Nurs 2004;104:40–51.
16. Bailes BK. Perioperative care of the elderly surgical patient. AORN J 2000;72:186–207.
17. Sadavoy J, Jarvik LF, Grossberg GT. Principles and practice of geriatric surgery. In: Rosenthal RA, editor. Comprehensive textbook of geriatric psychiatry. New York: Springer Publishing; 2004. p. 85–7, 281–308.
18. Changes with aging. Available at: http://www.ageworks.com/information_on_aging/changeswithaging/index.shtml. Accessed March 18, 2007.
19. What is normal aging? Available at: http://www.agingcarefl.org/aging/normalAging. Accessed March 10, 2007.
20. Cotter V, Smith C. Normal aging changes. Available at: http://www.geronurseonline.org/index.cfm?section_id=31&geriatric_topic_id=11&sub_section_id=77&page_id=166&tab=2. Accessed March 10, 2007.
21. Bailes BK. Hypothyroidism in elderly patients. AORN J 1999;69:1026–30.
22. Bailes BK. Hyperthyroidism in elderly patients. AORN J 1999;69:254–8.
23. Meiner S. Metabolic and endocrine problems. In: Meiner S, Luggen A, editors. NGNA core curriculum for gerontological nursing. 2nd edition. Philadelphia: Mosby Publishing; 2001. p. 111–3.
24. Dubin S. The physiologic changes of aging. Orthop Nurs 1992;11:45–50. Available at: http://www.cinahl.com/cgi-bin/refsvc?jid=295&;accno=1992147964.
25. Gomolin IH, Aung MM, WolfKlein G, et al. Older is colder: temperature range and variation in older

people. J Am Geriatr Soc 2005;53:2170–2. Available at: http://www.cinahl.com/cgi-bin/refsvc?jid=748&;accno=2009083765.
26. Gruenewald DA, Brodkin KI, et al. Changes of aging. Available at: http://faculty.washington.edu/dgruen/physiol.htm. Accessed March 17, 2007.
27. Means KM. Anatomy of aging. Phys Med Rehabil State Art Rev 1996;10:653–64. Available at: http://www.cinahl.com/cgi-bin/refsvc?jid=886&accno=1997033656.
28. Atkinson P. Cardiovascular problems. In: Luggen A, Meiner S, editors. NGNA core curriculum for gerontological nursing. 2nd edition. Philadelphia: Mosby Publishing; 2001. p. 54–64.
29. Meiner S. Respiratory problems. In: Luggen A, Meiner S, editors. 2nd edition. Philadelphia: Mosby Publishing; 2001. p. 64–5.
30. Ersan T. Perioperative management of the geriatric patient. The eMedicine clinical knowledge base. 2006; March 10, 2007. Available at: Inova Fairfax Hospital Medical Library. Accessed March 10, 2007.
31. Meiner S. Gastrointestinal problems. In: Luggen A, Meiner S, editors. NGNA core curriculum for gerontological nursing. 2nd edition. Philadelphia: Mosby Publishing; 2001. p. 74–81.
32. Beliveau MM, Multach M. Perioperative care for the elderly patient. Med Clin North Am 2003;87:273–89.
33. Bolognia JL. Aging skin. American Journal of Medicine 1995;98:99S–103S.
34. Mokdad AH, Giles WH, Bowman BA, et al. Changes in health behaviors among older Americans, 1990 to 2000. Public Health Rep 2004;119:356–61.
35. Reno B. Urinary and reproductive problems. In: Luggen A, Meiner S, editors. NGNA core curriculum for gerontological nursing. 2nd edition. Philadelphia: Mosby Publishing; 2001. p. 84–7.
36. Rosenthal RA. Urinary and reproductive problems. In: Luggen A, Meiner S, editors. NGNA core curriculum for gerontological nursing. 2nd edition. Philadelphia: Mosby Publishing; 2001. p. 84–7.
37. Fair WR, Couch J, Wehner N. Prostatic antibacterial factor: identity and significance. Urology 1976;7:169–77.
38. Palmer RM. Perioperative care of the elderly patient. Cleve Clin J Med 2006;73:S106–10.
39. Paynter D, Mamaril ME. Perianesthesia challenges in geriatric pain management. J Perianesth Nurs 2004;19:385–91.
40. Luggen A, Meiner S. Sensory problems. In: Luggen A, Meiner S, editors. Sensory problems. 2nd edition. Philadelphia: Mosby Publishing; 2001. p. 158–65.
41. Amella EJ. Decision making for tube feeding in dementia: when evidence becomes paramount. J Clin Nurs 2003;12:793–5.
42. Amella EJ. Resistance at mealtimes for persons with dementia. J Nutr Health Aging 2002;6:117–22.
43. Luggen A. Musculoskeletal problems. In: Luggen A, Meiner S, editors. NGNA core curriculum for gerontological nursing. 2nd edition. Philadelphia: Mosby Publishing; 2001. p. 103–5.
44. Bailes BK. Diabetes mellitus and its chronic complications. AORN J 2002;76:266–82.
45. Zapka JG, Hennessy W, Carter RE, et al. End-of-life communication and hospital nurses: an educational pilot. J Cardiovasc Nurs 2006;21:223–31.

Preoperative Evaluation and Risk Assessment for Elderly Thoracic Surgery Patients

Michael Jaklitsch, MD*, Sarah Billmeier, MD

KEYWORDS

- Elderly • Preoperative assessment • Lung cancer
- Thoracic surgery • Geriatric assessment

The US population is aging. With an increase in life expectancy to 77.8 years and an aging baby boomer population, the number of people in the United States aged more than 65 years is expected to double by 2040. Currently, 12.5% of the US population is over the age of 65 years, and this percentage is projected to increase to 20% by the year 2050.[1–3] Older patients increasingly present for consideration of thoracic surgery, and determining the best management for this group of patients will be a more frequent challenge in the future. Although elderly patients present with a spectrum of thoracic disease, both benign and malignant, patients with cancer comprise the largest and most studied subset of this population.

LUNG CANCER

Lung cancer is a disease of the elderly. The median age of diagnosis in the United States is 71 years, and over 65% of patients are diagnosed after age 65 years. National Cancer Institute statistics indicate that lung cancer remains the second most common cancer after breast cancer in women and prostate cancer in men. It is the leading cause of cancer mortality as shown in **Figs. 1** and **2**.[4,5] In 2008 an estimated 215,020 Americans will be diagnosed and 161,840 people will die of lung cancer. Over 100,000 lung cancer deaths will be in patients aged more than 65 years.[6]

Surgical resection for non–small cell lung cancer (NSCLC) offers the best chance for cure if the disease is detected in the early stages. Unfortunately, only 15% to 25% of patients have locally staged disease at diagnosis. O'Rourke and colleagues used a database of 22,874 patients to demonstrate that the percentage of patients with surgically resectable disease at diagnosis increases with age. The percentage of lung cancer patients with local disease increased from 15.3% of those aged 54 years or younger to 19.2% of those aged 55 to 64 years to 21.9% of those aged 65 to 74 years to 25.4% of those aged 75 years or older.[7] Data published from the Surveillance, Epidemiology, and End Results (SEER) database in 2005 analyzing a cohort of 14,555 patients with early stage NSCLC showed that the frequency of stage I disease increased from 79% in patients aged less than 65 years to 87% in patients aged 75 years or greater.[8] Although the elderly are at increased risk of developing lung cancer, a higher proportion present with potentially curable disease.

Additionally, multiple studies have shown that, in elderly patients, tumor histology is more likely to be squamous cell carcinoma.[9–11] Mery and colleagues's[8] analysis of the SEER database showed that the frequency of squamous cell carcinoma increased from 27% in patients less than 65 years old to 38% in patients 75 years and older, with parallel decreases in the frequency of adenocarcinoma from 61% to 50% in corresponding age groups, as depicted in **Fig. 3**. Squamous cell carcinomas are associated with a higher incidence

Division of Thoracic Surgery, Brigham and Women's Hospital, 75 Francis Street, Boston, MA 02115, USA
* Corresponding author.
E-mail address: mjaklitsch@partners.org (M. Jaklitsch).

Thorac Surg Clin 19 (2009) 301–312
doi:10.1016/j.thorsurg.2009.07.004
1547-4127/09/$ – see front matter

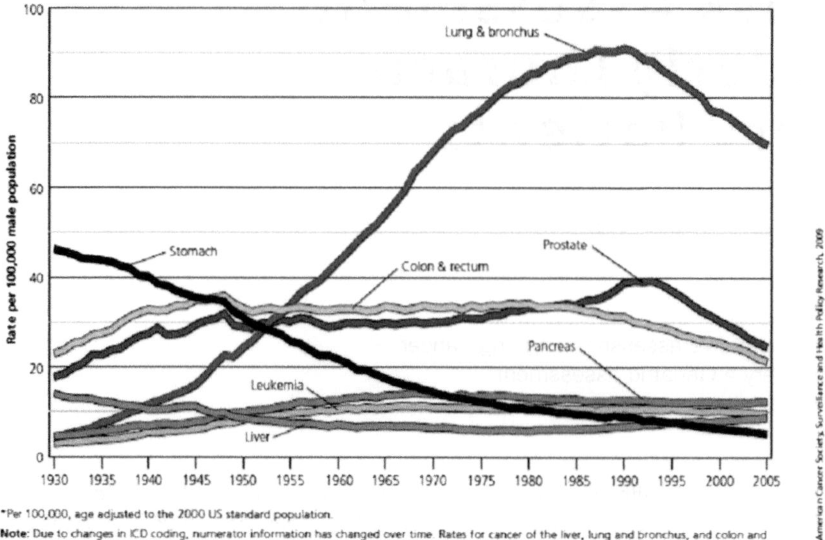

Fig. 1. Age-adjusted cancer death rates for males by site. (*From* American Cancer Society. Cancer Facts & Figures 2009. Atlanta: American Cancer Society; 2009; with permission.)

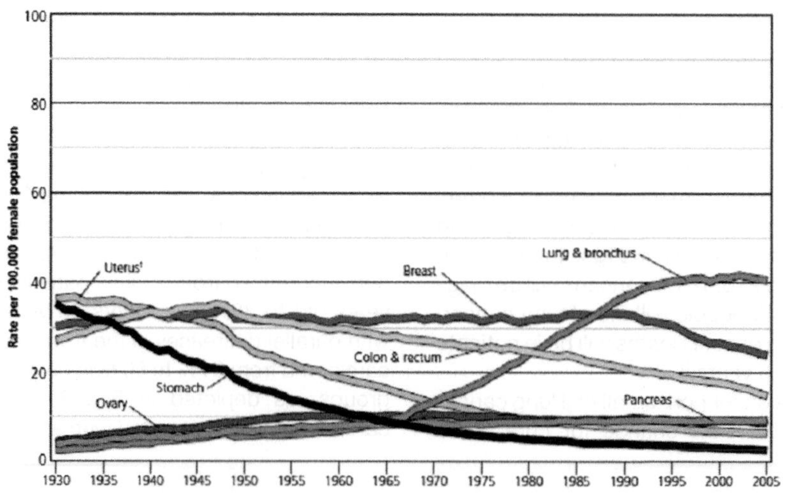

Fig. 2. Age-adjusted cancer death rates for females by site. (*From* American Cancer Society. Cancer Facts & Figures 2009. Atlanta: American Cancer Society; 2009; with permission.)

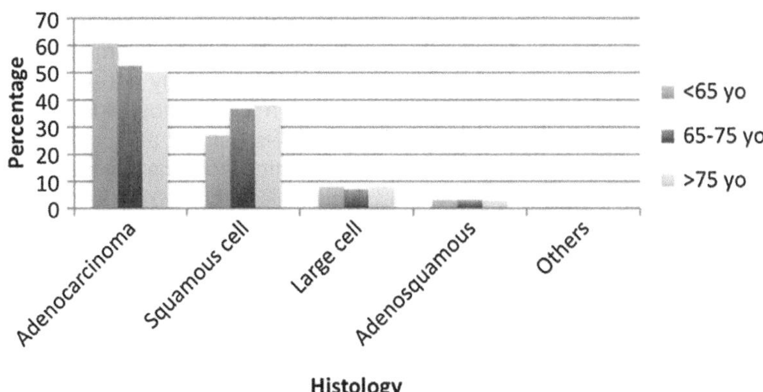

Fig. 3. Lung cancer histology by age. (*Data from* Mery CM, Pappas AN, Bueno R, et al. Similar long-term survival of elderly patients with non–small cell lung cancer treated with lobectomy or wedge resection within the Surveillance, Epidemiology, and End Results database. Chest 2005;128:237–45.)

of local disease,[7] tend to have lower recurrence rates, and may have longer survival times than non–squamous cell cancers.[12–14] Squamous cell tumors are more likely to be centrally located; therefore, they are more likely to require pneumonectomy for curative resection.

Lobectomy, removal of one of the five lobes of the lung and associated lymph nodes within a single pleural membrane, is considered the standard of care for surgical resection of early stage NSCLC.[8,15] Unfortunately, multiple studies substantiate age as a risk factor for death after thoracotomy. Using data from the 1960s and 1970s, several small single institution studies published operative mortality rates of 14% to 27% for the elderly depending on age and the type of surgery.[16–19] These findings were confirmed by a multi-institution prospective study by the Lung Cancer Study Group in 1983. Ginsberg and colleagues[20] reviewed 2200 cases of lung resection for cancer and found that operative mortality increased proportionally with age. Patients aged less than 60 years had a 1.3% 30-day mortality rate, with increasing rates of 4.1%, 7.0%, and 8.1% for the 60 to 69, 70 to 79, and 80 years or greater age groups, respectively.

More recently, Mery and colleagues determined the 30-day postoperative mortality rate for 14,555 patients who had undergone curative resections for treating stage I or II NSCLC over the period of 1992 to 1997. In an analysis of patients undergoing all types of surgery, there was a 0.45% mortality rate for those aged less than 65 years, a 0.6% rate for patients aged 65 to 74 years, and a 1.2% rate for patients aged 75 years or older (P = .001). Mortality differences were found to be primarily due to differences in the survival of patients undergoing lobectomy, with 0.3%, 0.5%, and 1.5% mortality rates, respectively, for these corresponding age groups (P = .0001). There was no statistically significant difference in perioperative mortality for patients of any age undergoing limited (wedge) resection.[21] Prior published reports likewise did not identify a difference in expected operative mortality after thoracotomy if lung-sparing operations were performed.[22–24]

The American College of Surgeons Oncology Group (ACOSOG) Z0030 Study published morbidity and mortality data in 2006 for 1023 clinically resectable T1 or T2, N0, or nonhilar N1 NSCLC patients randomized over a period from 1999 to 2004 to undergo lymph node sampling versus mediastinal lymph node dissection. Their age-stratified morbidity and mortality data are shown in **Table 1**. Notably, the overall mortality rate was 1.4%, improved from Ginsberg's reported rate of 3.8%, and was not statistically associated with age.[25] Ninety percent of patients in the ACOSOG Z0030 study underwent resection via a thoracotomy, with the remaining procedures performed as video-assisted thoracic surgery (VATS) or VATS-assisted resections. Operative mortality rates reported by Ginsberg for pneumonectomy and lobectomy were 6.2% and 2.9%, respectively, compared with 0% and 1.3% in the ACOSOG study. Notably, the pneumonectomy rate of the earlier study was 25.6% versus 4% in ACOSOG Z0030, partially explaining the higher mortality rate of the earlier study, leading to improved patient selection and greater use of parenchymal-sparing operations.

The operative risk of death after pulmonary resection is largely attributable to two anatomic disruptions: (1) loss of functional lung tissue and (2) the morbidity engendered by the access thoracotomy. Operative strategies tailored to the elderly

Table 1
ACOSOG Z0030 study age-stratified morbidity and mortality after resection for clinically resectable T1 or T2, N0, or non-hilar N1 non–small cell lung cancer

	Number of Patients Stratified by Age (%)				
Event	**<50 Years (n = 35)**	**50–59 Years (n = 171)**	**60–69 Years (n = 386)**	**70–79 Years (n = 361)**	**>80 Years (n = 70)**
One or more complications	8 (23)	50 (29)	136 (35)	162 (45)	34 (49)
Air leak >7 days	1 (3)	14 (8)	24 (6)	33 (9)	6 (9)
Chest tube drainage >7 days	0	14 (8)	42 (11)	53 (15)	9 (13)
Chylothorax	1 (3)	3 (2)	3 (1)	5 (1)	1 (1)
Hemorrhage	1 (3)	3 (2)	10 (3)	16 (4)	4 (6)
Recurrent nerve injury	0	0	5 (1)	2 (<1)	0
Atrial arrhythmia	1 (3)	13 (8)	53 (14)	68 (19)	12 (17)
Respiratory	4 (12)	8 (5)	30 (8)	29 (8)	3 (4)
Death	1 (2.6)	0	3 (0.8)	8 (2.2)	2 (2.9)

population have addressed both of these issues, with use of VATS to minimize the chest wall disruption of thoracotomy and consideration of limited resection for the most elderly.

VATS is defined as surgery performed through two or three incisions that are 2 cm in length. A utility incision less than 10 cm long may be used without spreading of the ribs. VATS procedures in the elderly have been shown to have lower morbidity and lower rates of postoperative delirium, and result in earlier ambulation, a lower narcotic requirement, and a quicker recovery time.[26–30] The extent of resection in elderly patients has been extensively debated, with several advocates for limited resections for the aged.

Multiple studies point to the undertreatment of cancer in the elderly, which is not limited to patients with lung cancer.[31] Published data from the SEER database show that the frequency of limited resection increases with age, with a decline of pneumonectomies and lobectomies with age. Approximately 30% of the most elderly patients in the database were denied surgery or were offered only palliative surgery, in contrast to 8% of the youngest patients.[8] Age is associated with declines in functional reserve and organ function, and optimal treatment is often affected by comorbid conditions. Adding to the complexity involved in treatment, the elderly have often not participated in clinical trials, forcing clinicians to rely primarily on retrospective data for treatment decisions.[32]

Using 2004 data, the life expectancy of an 80 year old in the United States is 9.1 years (8.2 years for males and 9.8 years for females), whereas the median survival for elderly patients with untreated early stage lung cancer is only 14 months.[33] This suggests that life limitation for an 80 year old with lung cancer is likely to be cancer related.[34] **Table 2** shows life table data from 2004 for patients older than 65 years.[35]

Despite improvements in mortality data over the past 2 decades, complication rates remain high, with rates approaching 50% in the eldest patients in the ACOSOG Z0030 study. Improvements in mortality statistics are likely multifactorial and reflect the result of global advancements in perioperative care ranging from improvements in anesthesia and intraoperative technique to specialized postoperative nursing. Perhaps most importantly, improvements in mortality may be related to better patient selection.

ESOPHAGEAL CANCER

Esophageal cancer likewise presents most commonly in elderly patients. Of the estimated

Table 2
Life expectancy by age (years), United States, 2004

Age	Total	Male	Female
65	18.7	17.1	20.0
70	15.1	13.7	16.2
75	11.9	10.7	12.8
80	9.1	8.2	9.8
85	6.8	6.1	7.2
90	5.0	4.4	5.2

16,000 patients diagnosed with esophageal cancer in the United States in 2008, approximately 60% were expected to be aged more than 65 years, with a median age at diagnosis of 69 years. The median age at death for patients with esophageal cancer during the time period from 2001 to 2005 was 70 years. Twenty-four percent of patients have localized cancer at the time of diagnosis.[6]

The survival rate for esophageal cancer is poor. Patients with surgically resectable tumors have a 5% to 30% 5-year survival rate.[36] The morbidity and mortality of surgery in conjunction with poor long-term survival after curative resection have made esophagectomy in elderly patients controversial, with multiple studies reporting high mortality and poor long-term survival.[37–39] Poon and colleagues published retrospective data comparing perioperative and long-term survival data in elderly versus younger patients and found a higher 30-day mortality in patients aged more than 70 years (7.2% versus 3.0%, $P = .02$) and worse long-term survival when deaths unrelated to comorbid conditions were included. Excluding unrelated medical condition deaths, long-term survival of younger and older patients was similar.[40] Because treatment programs that include esophagectomy are associated with the highest rates of cure, many authorities have concluded that surgery can be performed with acceptable risk in carefully selected elderly patients.[41,42]

Ellis and colleagues reported a retrospective analysis of 505 patients at a single institution over a 27-year period comparing patients aged more than 70 years with younger patients. There was a similar rate of resection with an insignificant increase in hospital mortality and similar morbidity between the two groups. The 5-year survival rate was 24.1% in elderly patients versus 22.4% in younger patients. Rates of symptom palliation were also similar between the two groups.[43] Elderly esophageal cancer patients should be carefully staged and risk stratified. Operative intervention should not be denied on the basis of age alone. Cardiopulmonary complications are the most frequent nonsurgical complications, and a preoperative evaluation should focus on optimization of these systems.

PHYSIOLOGIC CHANGES WITH AGE

Physiologic changes of the respiratory system associated with aging include reduced chest wall compliance with stiffening of calcified costal cartilages, diminished diaphragmatic excursion, and narrowing of the intervertebral disk space. A reduction of lung elastic recoil with loss of alveolar architecture produces a decreased alveolar gas exchange surface. Progressive atrophy creates weakness of the respiratory musculature. Additionally, a decrease in central nervous system responsiveness occurs. The loss of lung elastic recoil and decreased lung compliance diminishes negative intrapleural pressure, which prevents reopening of the small airways, resulting in air trapping and inadequate ventilation. Functionally, this manifests in a gradual decline of vital capacity and partial pressure of oxygen (P_{O2}), with an increased residual volume. The decline in motor power of the accessory muscles and stiffening of the chest wall also result in a declining forced expiratory volume in 1 second (FEV_1). Changes in lung compliance are not uniformly distributed; therefore, higher respiratory rates increase ventilation-perfusion mismatch. The elderly also exhibit a blunted ventilatory response to both hypoxic and hypercapneic insults.[44,45] Physiologic changes in lung mechanics make elderly patients particularly sensitive to narcotics and muscle relaxants, as well as to supine positioning. Additionally, elderly patients are at increased risk for respiratory tract infections due to waning immune responses.[46] Smoking in particular has been shown to cause bronchial mucociliary dysfunction,[47] which has been associated with increased susceptibility to infection.[48]

Increasing age is associated with declines in other organ systems as well. There is a decline in the glomerular filtration rate, an increased incidence of heart disease, and an increased incidence of cognitive dysfunction. Changes in body water composition decrease the volume of distribution of water-soluble drugs.[49] Additionally, elderly patients take more medications than younger patients and are vulnerable to adverse drug effects.

PREOPERATIVE EVALUATION

Elderly patients are at increased risk for preoperative morbidity and mortality due to comorbid conditions and a decreased ability to recover physiologic homeostasis after surgical stress, leading to the saying that, although elderly patients tolerate surgery, they do not tolerate the complications of surgery. Unfortunately, they are more prone to developing complications. Older patients represent a heterogeneous population. Some robust patients look younger than their stated age, whereas other frail patients look older than their stated age. The application of surgical therapy should be based on physiologic rather than chronologic age. A thorough preoperative assessment is imperative to determine whether a patient is an appropriate surgical candidate and to predict and avoid postoperative complications. Numerous risk assessment tools have been created to define preoperative variables that correlate with poor outcomes; however, an easy to use, strongly predictive tool has been elusive. Geriatric assessment tools aimed at predicting outcomes in the specific elderly surgical population remain under study.

All patients under consideration for thoracic surgery require a complete history and physical examination with particular attention to characterization of symptoms, smoking history, and weight loss. At a minimum, patients should undergo chest radiography, an electrocardiogram, a room air arterial blood gas and pulmonary function tests if undergoing lung resection, and basic laboratory work. Further work-up can be determined based on symptoms or the status of comorbid conditions. Accurate diagnosis and staging are of utmost importance to ensure that patients are appropriately chosen for operative resection.

Cardiac Risk Assessment

The American Heart Association (AHA) and American College of Cardiology (ACC) have published readily accessible consensus practice guidelines for perioperative cardiovascular evaluation for noncardiac surgery that provide a template for assessing patients of all ages.[50] The AHA/ACC guidelines describe a stepwise approach to preoperative assessment with risk stratification and further imaging determined by using symptoms, clinical predictors, and functional capacity. More recently in 2006, Auerbach and Goldman published a modification of the AHA/ACC guidelines[51] using the revised cardiac risk index (RCRI).[52] The RCRI was derived and validated by analyzing 4315 patients undergoing elective major noncardiac procedures. Six independent predictors of complications were identified and were included in the index: high risk surgery, a history of ischemic heart disease, a history of congestive heart failure, a history of cerebrovascular disease, preoperative treatment with insulin, and a preoperative creatinine level of greater than 2.0 mg/dL. Rates of major cardiac complications with zero, one, two, or three or more criteria were 0.5%, 1.3%, 4%, and 9%, respectively. The study included 1473 patients aged more than 70 years. Thoracic surgery was defined as high risk.

The clinical history should focus on an assessment for coronary risk factors and physical capacity, including the ability to climb two flights of stairs or walk one block. In general, patients with poor functional status, patients with one to two RCRI criteria, or patients with a history of angina or claudication should undergo noninvasive testing. In thoracic surgery patients, it may be difficult to determine if symptom etiology is the result of cardiac or pulmonary pathology; therefore, it is appropriate to have a low threshold for additional cardiac imaging and assessment by a cardiologist to assist with risk stratification.

Adrenergic modification with beta blockers in the perioperative period for thoracic surgery patients serves to reduce the risk of myocardial infarction and prevent postoperative supraventricular tachycardias. RCRI criteria have also been used to determine the need for perioperative beta blocker and statin therapy to prevent myocardial infarction or other cardiac complications. Patients with two or more RCRI criteria (thoracic surgery patients undergoing a resection by definition have at least one criteria) and no other long-term indications for beta blockade should still receive beta blockers at the time of surgery. Beta blockers should optimally continue for 1 month or indefinitely in patients with appropriate medical histories such as perioperative myocardial infarction.[51]

Supraventricular tachycardias are common after thoracic surgery, with a linear increase in risk as a function of age and baseline preoperative heart rate.[53] The risk of postoperative atrial fibrillation is 19% in patients undergoing lung resection for cancer.[54] Randomized trials of thoracic surgery patients have determined that calcium channel blockers or beta blockers can reduce the incidence of postoperative atrial fibrillation by 50% to 60%; however, beta blockers are associated with an increased risk of pulmonary edema. Neither class of medication reduces mortality. Three trials showed that digitalis increased the risk of atrial arrhythmias.[55] Beta blockers and calcium channel blockers will both reduce postoperative atrial fibrillation; however, beta blockers are generally preferred due to their broader benefits of cardiac risk reduction.

Pulmonary Risk Assessment

All patients undergoing lung resection surgery should have pulmonary function tests performed. The FEV_1 by spirometry is the most commonly measured value used to determine a patient's suitability for surgery. Data obtained in the 1970s from over 2000 patients showed a less than 5% mortality rate for patients with an FEV_1 greater than 1.5 L for lobectomy and greater than 2 L for pneumonectomy.[56,57] Absolute values for FEV_1 may create a bias against older people; however, a value of greater than 80% of predicted has been quoted by some as sufficient for a patient to undergo pneumonectomy without further pulmonary testing.[58] In reviewing more recent spirometry studies performed from 1994 to 2000, Datta and Lahiri concluded that, in NSCLC patients, increased postoperative morbidity and mortality were predicted by an FEV_1 of less than 2 L or less than 60% predicted for pneumonectomy, an FEV_1 of less than 1.6 L for lobectomy, and an FEV_1 of less than 0.6 L for wedge or segmentectomy.[59]

Lung resections have been undertaken in patients with much poorer lung function. In 2005 Linden and colleagues published data from a series of 100 consecutive patients with a preoperative FEV_1 of less than 35% of predicted undergoing lung tumor resection. In this series from an experienced academic center, mortality seems to have been positively affected by the recognition of and aggressive intervention to minimize the impact of morbid complications. There was a 1% mortality rate and a 36% complication rate. Furthermore, the pulmonary morbidities in this group of patients with tenuous lung function were sometimes life altering. Eleven patients were discharged with a new oxygen requirement, four patients experienced pneumonia, one patient became ventilator dependent, and three patients required intubation for more than 48 hours. Twenty-two percent of patients had prolonged air leaks.[60]

Ferguson and colleagues found that the preoperative diffusion capacity for carbon monoxide (DLCO) was more predictive of postoperative mortality than the FEV_1 in a study of 237 patients. In this study, a DLCO of less than 60% of predicted was associated with increased mortality, and a DLCO of less than 80% of predicted was predictive of increased pulmonary complications.[61] Other studies have not found this value to be a significant predictor of postoperative complications.[62,63] The DLCO and spirometry may be used as complimentary tests, particularly in patients with diffuse parenchymal disease or dyspnea that is out of proportion to the FEV_1, with a low DLCO prompting further evaluation.[57]

Formal and simple exercise testing evaluates the cardiopulmonary system under induced physiologic stress and has been found to be predictive of postoperative complications. Girish and colleagues prospectively studied symptom-limited stair climbing in patients undergoing thoracic and upper abdominal surgery. No complications occurred in patients who could climb seven flights of stairs, whereas 89% of patients unable to climb one flight of stairs had complications. Inability to climb two flights of stairs had a positive predictive value of 80%. The ability of patients to climb stairs was found to be inversely related to the length of postoperative hospital stay.[64] The 6-minute walk test (6MWT) measures the distanced walked over a period of 6 minutes. In a qualitative review, Solway concluded that the 6MWT was easy to administer and more reflective of activities of daily living (ADLs) than other walk tests.[65] Although stair climbing and the 6MWT are easy to perform, their use in elderly patients may be limited by orthopedic impairments, peripheral vascular insufficiency, or neurologic impairments.

As published previously,[66] the preoperative pulmonary evaluation for an elderly patient should consist of spirometry, the pulmonary DLCO, measurement of room air arterial blood gas, and exercise tolerance tests including stair climbing and the 6MWT. Patients with an FEV_1 greater than 1 L and no major abnormalities on other tests (FEV_1/FVC >50%, DLCO >50% predicted, arterial blood gas PaO_2 >45 mm Hg, tolerance of exercise tests) may safely proceed with surgery, including pneumonectomy (**Fig. 4**).

Further evaluation for patients who fall outside these criteria includes oxygen consumption (VO_2 max) testing and ventilation/perfusion scans to calculate predicted postoperative lung function. Measurement of maximal oxygen consumption (VO_2 max) by formal cardiopulmonary exercise testing is helpful to further risk stratify patients with borderline lung function. A VO_2 max of less than 10 mL/kg/min has been associated with a high operative morbidity (26% total in combined data) in several small case series. VO_2 max values of 10 to 15 mL/kg/min are associated with an intermediate perioperative morbidity (8.3% total), whereas patients with a value greater than 15 mL/kg/min can proceed with lung resection surgery with an acceptable mortality rate.[57]

Predicted postoperative lung function can be calculated by several methods such as anatomic estimation, ventilation or perfusion scans, or quantitative CT scans. The predicted

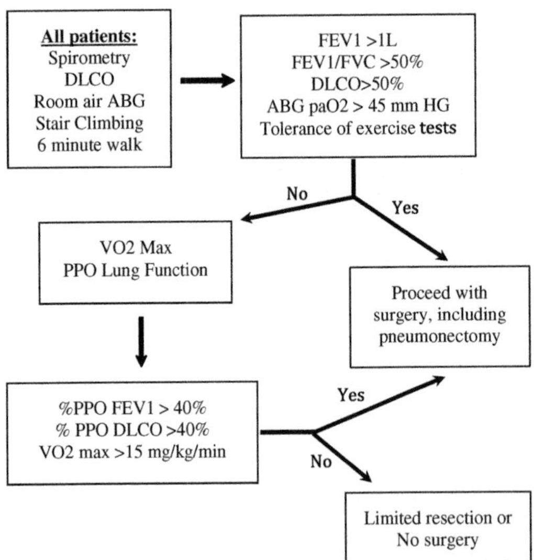

Fig. 4. Recommended pulmonary evaluation for patients undergoing lung resection surgery. ABG, arterial blood gas; DLCO, diffusion capacity for carbon monoxide; FEV_1, forced expiratory volume in 1 second; FVC, forced vital capacity; VO_2 max, maximal oxygen consumption; PPO, predicted postoperative.

postoperative FEV_1 ($ppoFEV_1$) by anatomic estimation is calculated by the following formula:

$$\text{ppoFEV1} = \text{preoperative FEV1} \times (1 - [\text{number of functional or unobstructed lung segments to be removed}/\text{total number of functional segments}])$$

For example, in a patient with a preoperative FEV_1 of 1.5 L without previous lung resection surgery undergoing a right upper lobectomy, the $ppoFEV_1$ would be calculated as 1.5 L $\times$ (1−3/19) = 1.25 L. In a patient with a previous left lower lobectomy with an FEV_1 of 1.5 L undergoing a right lower lobectomy, the $ppoFEV_1$ would be 1.5 L $\times$ (1 − 5/14) = 0.96 L. This equation is based on the 19 anatomic segments of the lung: five in the right lower lobe, five in the left lower lobe, two in the middle lobe, three in the right upper lobe, and four in the left upper lobe.

Using radionucleotide perfusion scanning, the postoperative FEV_1 is calculated by the following formula:

$$\text{Postoperative FEV1} = \text{preoperative FEV1} \times \%\ \text{of radioactivity contributed by nonoperated lung}$$

A $ppoFEV_1$ threshold of 0.8 L[67] or 0.7 L[68] has been suggested as a lower limit value for proceeding with lung resection. Absolute values of the $ppoFEV_1$ can underestimate postoperative lung in persons with a small stature or the elderly and can be converted into a percent-predicted postoperative (ppo%) lung function. Multiple studies have suggested that morbidity increases at a threshold $ppoFEV_1\%$ of less than 40 or a ppoDLCO% of less than 40.[61,69–72]

Cognitive and Functional Assessment

One of the most important pieces of information for an elderly patient is the likelihood of returning to baseline physical and mental function after surgery. Although patients and their families accept that there will be a postoperative recovery time in the hospital or rehabilitation setting, it is difficult to assess the magnitude of this functional decline and to predict the risk of permanent loss of independence. A paucity of data assess changes in quality of life after thoracic surgery in the elderly, and few studies have assessed whether surgery triggers postoperative loss of independence and a change in the need for assistance or living requirements. A study of 68 octogenarians undergoing pulmonary resection at the Johns Hopkins Medical Institutions showed that 80% of patients were discharged directly home from the hospital rather than to rehabilitation, offering some proxy information regarding immediate postoperative return to function.[73] Moller and colleagues[74] published a study in 1998 that showed a 25% rate of cognitive dysfunction at 1 week after operation from major noncardiac surgery in elderly patients (average age 68 years), with continued dysfunction in 9% at 3 months. Data from many studies verify a high incidence of postoperative cognitive dysfunction in the first week after surgery, and dysfunction tends to increase with age. Only one other study has substantiated long-term declines over controls, and some have suggested that the declines found in these studies may be due to random variation.[75,76] Kaneko and colleagues[77] determined that preoperative dementia was a risk factor for postoperative delirium. Furthermore, Fukuse and colleagues[78] found that thoracic surgery patients with preoperative dementia, as estimated by the mini-mental status examination (MMS), were fourfold more likely to have postoperative complications.

Geriatric Assessment

Several assessment indices have been applied to elderly patients to determine their risk for a poor outcome. Two assessment tools specifically aimed at oncogeriatric patients are under current study and are described herein.

The preoperative assessment of cancer in the elderly (PACE) is a tool designed by the International Society of Geriatric Oncology to assess the functional activities of oncogeriatric patients, with a goal of assessing the individualized surgical risk of these patients based on preoperative variables. Instruments used in PACE assessment include the MMS, Satariano's modified index of comorbidities, ADLs, instrumental activities of daily living (IADL), the Geriatric Depression Scale (GDS), the Brief Fatigue Inventory (BFI), the Eastern Cooperative Oncology Group (ECOG) performance status, the American Society of Anesthesiologists (ASA) score, and the Physiologic and Operative Severity Score for the enUmeration of Mortality and Morbidity (POSSUM) and Portsmouth (P)-POSSUM score. Preliminary data analyzing PACE components have been published, assessing 30-day morbidity rates in 215 patients with a median age of 76 years who underwent surgery for breast cancer (142 patients), urogenital cancer, colorectal cancer, gastroesophageal cancer, head and neck cancer, and gynecologic cancers. In the interim results, two components of PACE were associated with 30-day morbidity. Lower performance status and a lower ADL score were both associated with postoperative complications. The MMS, GDS, BFI, and ASA were not related to 30-day morbidity.[79] Further study with a larger sample size is ongoing.

The preliminary PACE results are consistent with prior studies that correlate preoperative functional and performance status with postoperative morbidity. Functional status describes the ability to perform self-care, self-maintenance, and physical activities. Traditional measures used to assess functional status are ADLs and IADLs. ADLs are six basic self-care skills, including the ability to bathe, dress, go to the toilet, transfer from a bed to chair, maintain continence, and feed one's self. IADLs include higher functioning skills that are used to maintain independence in the community. This scale assesses the ability to use the telephone, go shopping, prepare food, perform housekeeping and laundry, use various modes of transportation, assume responsibility for medications, and handle finances. Need for assistance in these tasks has been predictive of a prolonged hospital stay, nursing home placement, and home care requirements.[80,81] Poor nutritional status, defined as a body mass index (BMI) less than 22 kg/m^2 has been associated with an increased need for assistance with ADLs and decreased 1-year survival.[82]

Performance status is a standardized scale designed to measure the ability of a cancer patient to perform ordinary tasks. There are two scales—the Karnofsky performance scale that ranges from 0 (dead) to 100 (normal) and the ECOG scale that ranges from 0 (asymptomatic) to 5 (dead). Comparisons of the two scales have been validated with a large sample of patients.[83] Performance status has been used to select patients for entry into chemotherapy trials; however, it is also well accepted to be associated with postoperative morbidity.[84–86]

A thoracic surgery specific geriatric assessment is also under current study. This development protocol will assess the feasibility of using a baseline geriatric assessment of presurgical patients with lung nodules to determine whether components of the assessment can predict the choice of operative procedure or the trajectory of functional recovery. This study aims to determine which scales have the greatest predictive value for postoperative morbidity, mortality, length of stay, and the need for allied health services.[87] This study protocol uses some of the same components as PACE but adds elements that are specific to thoracic surgery. Preoperatively, this study will assess scales of functional status, comorbidity, cognition, psychologic status, social function and support, nutritional status, and the lung function BODE index, which includes BMI, spirometry, the Cancer Dyspnea Scale, and a 6-minute walk.

SUMMARY

Assessment for thoracic surgery in elderly patients should proceed on the basis of physiologic rather than chronologic age. Thoracic surgery has been shown to be safe in selected elderly patients, and age should not be a contraindication to a therapy that offers the best chance of cure for early stage cancer patients. A targeted preoperative assessment can help individualize the morbidity and mortality risk of surgery for each patient and provide the surgeon and patient with the information needed for operative decision making. Operative interventions in the elderly require coordinated attention to the specific requirements of the aged. Specialized multidisciplinary care provided by primary care physicians, geriatric specialists, cardiologists, oncologists, surgeons, anesthesia personnel, nurses, physical therapists, and nutritionists will optimize care for the elderly thoracic surgery patient. Careful selection of patients for surgery has contributed to the improvement in operative mortality over time, and refinements in preoperative testing should continue this trend in the future.

REFERENCES

1. Kung HC, Hoyery DL, Xu J. Deaths: final data for 2005. Centers for Disease Control. Natl Vital Stat Rep 2008;56(10):1–120.
2. US Census Bureau, population division. Table 2. Projections of the population by selected age groups and sex for the United States: 2010 to 2050 (NP2008–T2). Release date August 14, 2008. Available at: http://www.census.gov/population/www/projections/files/nation/summary/np2008-t2.xls. Accessed September 2, 2009.
3. US Census Bureau, population division. Table 3. Percent distribution of the projected population by selected age groups and sex for the United States: 2010 to 2050 (NP2008–T3). Release date August 14, 2008. Available at: http://www.census.gov/population/www/projections/files/nation/summary/np2008-t3.xls. Accessed September 2, 2009.
4. American Cancer Society. Cancer facts & figures: age-adjusted cancer death rates, males by site. Available at: http://www.cancer.org/docroot/MED/content/MED_1_1_Most_Requested_Graphs_and_Figures_2008.asp. 2008. Accessed September 2, 2009.
5. American Cancer Society. Cancer facts & figures: age-adjusted cancer death rates, females by site. Available at: http://www.cancer.org/docroot/MED/content/MED_1_1_Most_Requested_Graphs_and_Figures_2008.asp. 2008. Accessed September 2, 2009.
6. Ries LAG, Melbert D, Krapcho M, et al. SEER cancer statistics review, 1975–2005. Bethesda (MD): National Cancer Institute. Available at: http://seer.cancer.gov/csr/1975_2005. Based on November 2007 SEER data submission posted to the SEER Web site, 2008. Accessed September 2, 2009.
7. O'Rourke MA, Feussner JR, Feigl P, et al. Age trends of lung cancer stage at diagnosis: implications for lung cancer screening in the elderly. JAMA 1987; 258:921–6.
8. Mery CM, Pappas AN, Bueno R, et al. Similar long-term survival of elderly patients with non–small cell lung cancer treated with lobectomy or wedge resection within the Surveillance, Epidemiology, and End Results database. Chest 2005;128:237–45.
9. Teeter SM, Holmes FF, McFarlane MJ. Lung carcinoma in the elderly population: influence of histology on the inverse relationship of stage to age. Cancer 1987;60:1331–6.
10. Weinmann M, Jeremie B, Toomes H, et al. Treatment of lung cancer in the elderly. Part I. Non–small cell lung cancer. Lung Cancer 2003;39:233–53.
11. Morandi U, Stefani A, Golinelli M, et al. Results of surgical resection in patients over the age of 70 years with non–small cell lung cancer. Eur J Cardiothorac Surg 1997;11:432–49.
12. Gail MH, Eagan RT, Feld R, et al. Prognostic factors in patients with resected stage I non–small cell lung cancer: a report from the Lung Cancer Study Group. Cancer 1984;54:1802–13.
13. Mountain CF, Lukeman JM, Hammar SP, et al. Lung cancer classification: the relationship of disease extent and cell type to survival in a clinical trials population. J Surg Oncol 1987;35:147–56.
14. Deslauriers J, Gregoire J. Surgical therapy of early non–small cell lung cancer. Chest 2000; 117(Suppl):104S–9S.
15. Faulkner SL. Is lobectomy the gold standard for stage I lung cancer in year 2000? [abstract]. Chest 2000;118(Suppl 4):119S.
16. Bates M. Results of surgery for bronchial carcinoma in patients aged 70 and over. Thorax 1970;25:77–8.
17. Evans EW. Resection of bronchial carcinoma in the elderly. Thorax 1973;28:86–8.
18. Kirsh MM, Rotman H, Bove E, et al. Major pulmonary resection for bronchial carcinoma in the elderly. Ann Thorac Surg 1976;22:369–73.
19. Harviel JD, McNamara JJ, Straehley CJ. Surgical treatment of lung cancer in patients over the age of 70 years. J Thorac Cardiovasc Surg 1978;75:802–5.
20. Ginsberg RJ, Hill LD, Eagan RT, et al. Modern thirty-day operative mortality for surgical resections in lung cancer. J Thorac Cardiovasc Surg 1983;86:654–8.
21. Mery CM, Jaklitch MT. Lung resection in the elderly, correspondence. Chest 2006;129:496–7.
22. Albano WA. Should elderly patients undergo surgery for cancer. Geriatrics 1977;32:105–8.
23. Breyer RH, Zippe C, Pharr WF, et al. Thoracotomy in patients over age seventy years: ten-year experience. J Thorac Cardiovasc Surg 1981;81:187–93.
24. Zapatero J, Madrigal L, Lago J, et al. Thoracic surgery in the elderly: review of 100 cases. Acta Chir Hung 1990;31:227–34.
25. Allen MS, Darling GE, Pechet TT, et al. ACOSOG Z0030 Study Group. Morbidity and mortality of major pulmonary resections in patients with early stage lung cancer: initial results of the randomized, prospective ACOSOG Z0030 trial. Ann Thorac Surg 2006;81(3):1013–9.
26. Decamp MM Jr, Jaklitsch MT, Mentzer SJ, et al. The safety and versatility of video-thoracoscopy: a prospective analysis of 895 cases. J Am Coll Surg 1995;181:113–20.
27. McKenna R. Thoracoscopic lobectomy with mediastinal sampling in 80 year old patients. Chest 1994; 106:1902–4.
28. Landreneau RL, Sugarbaker DJ, Mack MJ, et al. Postoperative pain-related morbidity: video-assisted thoracic surgery versus thoracotomy. Ann Thorac Surg 1993;56:1285–9.
29. Jaklitsch MT, Bueno R, Swanson SJ, et al. Video-assisted thoracic surgery in the elderly: a review of 307 cases. Chest 1996;110:751–8.

30. Cattaneo SM, Park BJ, Wilton AS, et al. Use of video-assisted thoracic surgery for lobectomy in the elderly results in fewer complications. Ann Thorac Surg 2008;85:231–6.
31. Samet J, Hunt WC, Key C, et al. Choice of cancer therapy varies with age of patient. JAMA 1986;255: 3385–90.
32. Gridelli C, Langer C, Maione P, et al. Lung cancer in the elderly. J Clin Oncol 2007;25(14):1899–907.
33. McGarry RC, Song G, des Rosiers P, et al. Observation-only management of early stage, medically inoperable lung cancer: poor outcome. Chest 2002;121:1155–8.
34. Yellin A, Brenfield JR. Surgery for bronchogenic carcinoma in the elderly. Am Rev Respir Dis 1985; 131:197.
35. Arias E. United States life tables, 2004. Natl Vital Stat Rep 2007;56(9):1–39.
36. Kelsen DP, Bains M, Burt M. Neoadjuvant chemotherapy and surgery of cancer of the esophagus. Semin Surg Oncol 1990;6(5):268–73.
37. Ferguson MK, Martin TR, Reeder LB, et al. Mortality after esophagectomy: risk factor analysis. World J Surg 1997;23:599–604.
38. Adam DJ, Craig SR, Sang CT, et al. Esophagectomy for carcinoma in the octogenarian. Ann Thorac Surg 1996;61:190–4.
39. Suglmachi K, Matsuzaki K, Matsuura H, et al. Evaluation of surgical treatment of carcinoma of the oesophagus in the elderly: 20 years experience. Br J Surg 1985;72:28–32.
40. Poon RT, Law SY, Chu KM, et al. Esophagectomy for carcinoma of the esophagus in the elderly: results of current surgical management. Ann Surg 1998; 227(3):357–64.
41. Kinugasa S, Tachibana M, Yoshimura H, et al. Esophageal resection in elderly esophageal carcinoma patients: improvement in postoperative complications. Ann Thorac Surg 2001;71:414–8.
42. Thomas P, Doddoli C, Neville P, et al. Esophageal cancer resection in the elderly. Eur J Cardiothorac Surg 1996;10:941–6.
43. Ellis FH Jr, Williamson WA, Heatley GJ. Cancer of the esophagus and cardia: does age influence treatment selection and surgical outcomes. J Am Coll Surg 1998;187(4):345–51.
44. Rossi A, Ganassini A, Tantucci C, et al. Aging and the respiratory system. Aging (Milano) 1996;8(3):143–61.
45. Janssens JP, Pache JC, Nicod LP. Physiological changes in respiratory function associated with ageing. Eur Respir J 1999;13:197–205.
46. Meyer KC. Lung infections and aging. Ageing Res Rev 2004;3(1):55–67.
47. Verra F, Escudier E, Lebargy F, et al. Ciliary abnormalities in bronchial epithelium of smokers, ex-smokers, and nonsmokers. Am J Respir Crit Care Med 1995;151(3):630–4.
48. Salathe M, O'Riordan TG, Wanner A. Treatment of mucociliary dysfunction. Chest 1996;110:1048–57.
49. McLesky CH. Anesthesia for the geriatric patient. In: Barash PG, Cullen BF, Staelting RK, editors. Clinical anesthesia. 2nd edition. Philadelphia: JB Lippincott; 1992. p. 1353–83.
50. Eagle KA, Berger PB, Calkins H, et al. ACC/AHA guideline update for perioperative cardiovascular evaluation for noncardiac surgery. Circulation 2002;105:1257–67.
51. Auerbach A, Goldman L. Assessing and reducing the cardiac risk of noncardiac surgery. Circulation 2006;113:1361–76.
52. Lee TH, Marcantonio MD, Mangione CM, et al. Derivation and prospective validation of a simple index for prediction of cardiac risk of major noncardiac surgery. Circulation 1999;100:1043–9.
53. Passman RS, Gingold DS, Amar D, et al. Prediction rule for atrial fibrillation after major noncardiac thoracic surgery. Ann Thorac Surg 2005;79:1698–703.
54. Roselli EE, Murthy SC, Rice TW, et al. Atrial fibrillation complicating lung cancer resection. J Thorac Cardiovasc Surg 2005;130:438–44.
55. Sedrakyan A, Treasure T, Browne J, et al. Pharmacologic prophylaxis for postoperative atrial tachyarrhythmia in general thoracic surgery: evidence from randomized clinical trials. J Thorac Cardiovasc Surg 2005;129:997–1005.
56. British Thoracic Society, Society of Cardiothoracic Surgeons of Great Britain and Ireland Working Party. Guidelines on the selection of patients with lung cancer for surgery. Thorax 2001;56:89–108.
57. Colice GL, Shafazand S, Griffin JP, et al. Physiologic evaluation of the patient with lung cancer being considered for resectional surgery: ACCP evidence-based clinical practice guidelines [2nd edition]. Chest 2007;132:161–77.
58. Wyser C, Stulz P, Soler M, et al. Prospective evaluation of an algorithm for the functional assessment of lung resection candidates. Am J Respir Crit Care Med 1999;159:1450–6.
59. Datta D, Lahiri B. Preoperative evaluation of patients undergoing lung resection surgery. Chest 2003;123: 2096–103.
60. Linden PA, Bueno R, Colson YL, et al. Lung resection in patients with preoperative FEV1 <35% predicted. Chest 2005;127:1984–90.
61. Ferguson MK, Little L, Rizzo L, et al. Diffusing capacity predicts morbidity and mortality after pulmonary resection. J Thorac Cardiovasc Surg 1988;96:894–900.
62. Stephan F, Boucheseiche S, Hollande J, et al. Pulmonary complications following lung resection: a comprehensive analysis of incidence and possible risk factors. Chest 2000;118:1263–70.
63. Botsen PC, Block AJ, Moulder PC. Relationship between preoperative pulmonary function tests

and complications after thoracotomy. Surg Gynecol Obstet 1981;52:813–5.

64. Girish M, Trayner E, Dammann O, et al. Symptom-limited stair climbing as a predictor of postoperative cardiopulmonary complications after high risk surgery. Chest 2001;120:1147–51.
65. Solway S, Brooks D, Lacasses Y, et al. A qualitative systematic overview of the measurement properties of functional walk tests used in the cardiorespiratory domain. Chest 2001;119(1):256–70.
66. Jaklitsch MT, Mery CM, Audisio RA. The use of surgery to treat lung cancer in elderly patients. Lancet Oncol 2003;4:463–71.
67. Olsen GN, Block AJ, Tobias JA. Prediction of post-pnemonectomy pulmonary function using quantitative macroaggregate lung scanning. Chest 1974; 66:13–6.
68. Pate P, Tenholder MF, Griffin JP, et al. Preoperative assessment of the high-risk patient for lung resection. Ann Thorac Surg 1996;61:1494–500.
69. Markos J, Mullan BP, Hillman DR, et al. Preoperative assessment as a predictor of mortality and morbidity after lung resection. Am Rev Respir Dis 1989;139: 902–10.
70. Bolliger CT, Wyser C, Boser H, et al. Lung scanning and exercise testing for the prediction of postoperative performance in lung resection candidates at increased risk of complications. Chest 1995;108: 341–8.
71. Holden DA, Rice TW, Stefmach K, et al. Exercise testing, 6-min walk, and stair climb in the evaluation of patients at high risk for pulmonary resection. Chest 1992;102:1774–9.
72. Wahi R, McMurtry MJ, DeCaro LF, et al. Determinants of perioperative morbidity and mortality after pneumonectomy. Ann Thorac Surg 1989;48: 33–7.
73. Brock MV, Kim MP, Hooker CM, et al. Pulmonary resection in octogenarians with stage I non–small cell lung cancer: a 22-year experience. Ann Thorac Surg 2004;77:271–7.
74. Moller JT, Cluitmans P, Rasmussen LS, et al. Long-term postoperative cognitive dysfunction in the elderly: ISPOCD1 study. Lancet 1998;351:857–61.
75. Rasmussen LS, Siersma VD, ISPOCD Group. Postoperative cognitive dysfunction: true deterioration versus random variation. Acta Anaesthesiol Scand 2004;48:1137–43.
76. Newman S, Stygall J, Shaefi S, et al. Postoperative cognitive dysfunction after noncardiac surgery. Anesthesiology 2007;106:572–90.
77. Kaneko T, Takahashi S, Naka T, et al. Postoperative delirium following gastrointestinal surgery in elderly patients. Surg Today 1997;27:107–11.
78. Fukuse T, Satoda N, Hijiya K, et al. Importance of a comprehensive geriatric assessment in prediction of complications following thoracic surgery in elderly patients. Chest 2005;127:886–91.
79. Audisio RA, Ramesh H, Longo W, et al. Preoperative assessment of surgical risk in oncogeriatric patients. Oncologist 2005;10:262–8.
80. Narian O, Rubenstein L, Wieland B, et al. Predictors of immediate and 6 month outcomes in hospitalized elderly patients: the importance of functional status. J Am Geriatr Soc 1988;36:775–83.
81. Reuben D, Rubenstein L, Hirsch SH, et al. Value of functional status as a predictor of mortality: results of a prospective study. Am J Med 1992;93(6):663–9.
82. Landi F, Zaccala G, Gambassi G, et al. Body mass index and mortality among older people living in the community. J Am Geriatr Soc 1999;47:1072.
83. Buccheri G, Ferrigno D, Tamburini M. Karnofsky and ECOG performance status scoring in lung cancer: a prospective, longitudinal study of 536 patients from a single institution. Eur J Cancer 1996;32(7):1135–41.
84. Harpole DH Jr, Herndon JF 2nd, Young WG Jr, et al. Stage I non–small cell lung cancer: a multivariate analysis of treatment methods and patterns of recurrence. Cancer 1995;76:787–96.
85. Stamatis G, Djuric D, Eberhardt W, et al. Postoperative morbidity and mortality after induction chemoradiotherapy for locally advanced lung cancer: an analysis of 350 operated patients. Eur J Cardiothorac Surg 2002;22:292–7.
86. Ferguson MK, Vigneswaran WT. Diffusing capacity predicts morbidity after lung resection in patients without obstructive lung disease. Ann Thorac Surg 2008;85(4):1158–64.
87. Jaklitsch MT, Battafarano R, Hurria A. CALGB protocol proposal: a study to compare surgical choice and recovery as predicted by a brief geriatric assessment for patients 70 years of age and older undergoing surgical resection for lung nodules. Unpublished study protocol, used with permission.

Benign Thoracic Disease in the Elderly

Rita A. Mukhtar, MD, Pierre R. Theodore, MD*

KEYWORDS

• Benign • Pulmonary disease • Elderly • Nodules
• Thoracic surgery • Chest

Elderly patients present challenges in diagnosis and treatment of various disease processes. Although they may develop thoracic diseases seen in other age groups, older patients often have atypical presentations of these diseases, and may be vulnerable to thoracic pathology as a result of comorbid diseases. Pulmonary function testing of the elderly population shows increased ventilation-perfusion mismatch, decreased forced expiratory volumes, and decreased diffusion capacities. Combined with increased chest wall rigidity, decreasing muscle mass, impaired mucociliary clearance, blunted perception of dyspnea, and possible increased aspiration risk because of underlying neurologic dysfunction, these physiologic changes associated with aging make this population particularly vulnerable to thoracic disease.[1]

DISEASE OF THE CHEST WALL AND PLEURA

Mondor's Disease

Mondor's disease is a benign thrombophlebitis usually involving the thoracoepigastric and lateral thoracic veins. Three fourths of patients are women. Although the anterior and lateral chest wall are most commonly affected, Mondor's disease has been reported in the antecubital fossa, inguinal region, axilla, penis, abdomen, and lower limbs.[2]

The pathogenesis involves formation of venous thrombi, with resultant venous occlusion and fibrosis. The overlying skin retracts, creating characteristic cordlike structures, often starting from the areola or axilla. Although the etiology is unknown, there is an association with hypercoagulable states, thoracic surgical procedures, breast infections, hyperextension of the upper extremity, and intravenous drug abuse. Patients typically present with localized chest pain, and palpable cords on the chest wall. Although Mondor's disease itself is a benign, self-limited disease, it has been associated with the presence of carcinoma of the breast.

Treatment involves local application of heat, systemic or topical nonsteroidal anti-inflammatories, and rest of the affected limb. Pain usually resolves in about 10 days, whereas skin changes may take longer to resolve. For chronic or subacute cases, resection of the thrombotic vessels can be considered. There is no clear benefit of anticoagulation.

Lung Herniation

Lung herniation results when the lung parenchyma and pleural membranes protrude through a defect in the thoracic wall. It can result from congenital abnormalities, trauma, underlying disease, or thoracic surgical procedures. Spontaneous lung herniation secondary to vigorous coughing or playing a wind instrument has been reported.[3] Patients may be asymptomatic, or present with a bulge on the chest wall, hemoptysis owing to strangulation of herniated lung, or recurrent pulmonary infections. In patients undergoing minimally invasive thoracic surgery, the anterior approach appears to have a higher incidence of postoperative lung hernia development, likely because of inherent weakness in the thoracic cage where there is only a single layer of intercostal muscles.[4]

Department of Surgery, University of California, San Francisco, 1600 Divisadero Street, Box 1724, San Francisco, CA 94115, USA
* Corresponding author.
E-mail address: Pierre.Theodore@ucsfmedctr.org (P.R. Theodore).

Thorac Surg Clin 19 (2009) 313–319
doi:10.1016/j.thorsurg.2009.07.001
1547-4127/09/$ – see front matter

thoracic.theclinics.com

Predisposing factors for lung herniation include chronic obstructive pulmonary disease, inflammatory or neoplastic processes, and chronic steroid use. Lung herniation is unlikely to recover spontaneously, but surgical treatment is not mandatory for all lung hernias. Indications for operative intervention include strangulated lung, hemoptysis, and pain. Some authors advocate repair for all anterior hernias, even if asymptomatic, to avoid extension into the abdominal wall. Surgical treatment involves identification of the hernia sac, freeing the lung from adhesions, and patch repair. Minimally invasive repairs with videoscopic techniques have been described.

Pneumomediastinum

The primary development of free air in the mediastinum, or spontaneous pneumomediastinum, must be distinguished from secondary pneumomediastinum, as the two processes have very different clinical implications. Spontaneous pneumomediastinum results from a sudden increase in intrathoracic pressure, leading to increased intra-alveolar pressure. Alveolar rupture then allows air to track along the bronchovascular tissue sheath toward the mediastinum.[5]

The most common cause of spontaneous pneumomediastinum is forceful emesis, although intense coughing, screaming, childbirth, and bronchospasm have been reported as causative events. Predisposing factors include asthma and idiopathic pulmonary fibrosis. Patients can present with chest pain, shortness of breath, subcutaneous emphysema, or Hammon's sign, crepitus heard with the heart beat on auscultation of the chest.

Spontaneous pneumomediastinum is a benign condition for which treatment is usually expectant. The diagnosis of spontaneous pneumomediastinum is one of exclusion however, and the presence of free air on chest radiographs mandates differentiation from secondary pneumomediastinum. By contrast, secondary pneumomediastinum, which results most commonly from blunt or penetrating trauma, interventions in the esophagus or tracheobronchial tree, or infectious processes, is associated with life-threatening injury to the aerodigestive tract and carries a high mortality rate.

Kyphosis

Kyphosis is a common problem, and may contribute to pulmonary dysfunction in the elderly. It is an exaggerated posterior convexity of the thoracic spine, which increases with aging. This spinal deformity results from the combined effects of osteoporotic vertebral fractures, arthritis, intervertebral disk thinning, and reduced muscular tone. Vertebral compression fractures are estimated to occur in one third of women older than 65 years, and half of women older than 80. One study found that more than 80% of patients older than 80 had kyphosis.[6]

As with younger patients with spinal deformities, older patients with kyphosis suffer increased mortality from pulmonary disease, and measurable differences in spirometric evaluation. Women with radiographically evident vertebral fractures have double the mortality from pulmonary causes compared with women without vertebral fractures. Additionally, severe kyphosis is strongly predictive of pulmonary death.

Kyphosis resulting from osteoporotic vertebral fractures is thought to result in pulmonary impairment, resulting in a restrictive pattern evident in pulmonary function testing. In one study, kyphotic participants reported more dyspnea, and had restrictive and obstructive ventilatory patterns on spirometric testing.[7] With worsening kyphosis, or a Cobb's angle greater than 55 degrees, impairment is considerable. Cobb's angle is calculated by drawing lines parallel to the vertebral body at the superior aspect of the spinal curvature and the vertebral body at the inferior aspect of the spinal curvature, and then measuring the angle formed by the intersection of two lines perpendicular to these.

After kyphoplasty, forced vital capacity and maximum voluntary ventilation have been shown to improve. It is unclear whether this is related to improved pain or improved pulmonary mechanics. Difficulties in interpretation of existing studies include inconsistencies in methods used to measure height and kyphosis, as well as variability in tested pulmonary function parameters. However, given its high prevalence and association with poor pulmonary outcomes, kyphosis may be an underrecognized contributor to dyspnea in the elderly population.[8]

NEOPLASTIC DISEASE

Benign Lung Tumors

Benign neoplasms of the lung are uncommon tumors. Either epithelial or mesenchymal in origin, they can present with cough, pneumonia, hemoptysis, or be completely asymptomatic. In asymptomatic patients, the use of diagnostic imaging techniques identifies these lesions, often resulting in their resection for diagnostic purposes. Lack of progression of a pulmonary lesion over a minimum of 2 years is required to radiographically rule out a malignant process. Reviews of surgical series of patients with benign lung tumors show hamartomas to be the most prevalent. The age range is wide, with most benign tumors of adulthood presenting at a median age of 52 years. Various epithelial and mesenchymal benign neoplasms are described in the following paragraphs (**Table 1**).[9,10]

Epithelial tumors

Papillomas Papillomas occasionally occur in the lower airway. These are generally exophytic tumors, affecting men more often than women, and children most commonly. Papillomas have been classified as squamous, glandular, and mixed. Squamous papillomas are associated with human papilloma virus (HPV), whereas the more rare glandular papillomas are not. Squamous papillomas are thought to result from ororespiratory HPV exposure during vaginal delivery. As with other lesions caused by HPV infection, those papillomas caused by high-risk strains of the virus are at risk for malignant transformation to squamous carcinoma.[11]

Papillomas often present as thin-walled cysts and nodules with postobstructive atelectasis on chest radiograph. Histologically, exophytic papillomas have an epithelial layer covering a central fibrovascular core that protrudes into the airway lumen. Stratified squamous epithelium lines the squamous papillomas, whereas a single layer of columnar nonciliated epithelial cells line the glandular papillomas.

Recurrent respiratory papillomatosis is managed by endoscopic cryotherapy, laser, or microdebrider treatment. Attempts at management with transforming growth factor–beta cytokine blockade have met with some success in younger patients, but most are managed local ablative techniques rather than systemic therapy.

Sclerosing hemangioma (pneumocytoma) Benign lung neoplasms with a female predominance, these lesions are thought to arise from type II pneumocytes. They are well-circumscribed, containing two morphologic populations, cuboidal epithelium resembling type II pneumocytes, and round to oval stromal cells.

Alveolar adenoma Alveolar adenomas are unusual neoplasms typically found in the lung periphery with no gender predilection. They are usually identified as solitary asymptomatic pulmonary nodules in adults, and classified as epithelial neoplasms, although mesenchymal origin has also been suggested.

Table 1
Benign tumors of the lower respiratory tract, World Health Organization classification 2004[10]

Epithelial	Mesenchymal	Miscellaneous	Tumorlike Conditions
Papilloma	Hamartoma	Thymoma	Minute meningothelial nodules
Squamous	Localized fibrous tumor	Mature teratoma	Nodular lymphoid hyperplasia
Glandular	Chondroma	—	Inflammatory pseudotumor
Mixed	Leiomyoma	—	Localized organizing pneumonia
Sclerosing hemangioma	Lipoma	—	Nodular amyloid
Alveolar adenoma	Clear cell tumor	—	Hyalinizing granuloma
Papillary adenoma	Other soft tissue tumors	—	Bronchial inflammatory polyp
Mucous gland adenoma	—	—	Micronodular penumocyte hyperplasia
Pleomorphic adenoma	—	—	Endometriosis
Mucinous cystadenoma	—	—	Others—rounded atelectasis and congenital lesions

Type II pneumocyte papilloma These are rare, benign neoplasms composed of type II pneumocyte-lined papillae. They are typically solitary, well-circumscribed lesions in the periphery.

Mucous gland adenomas Mucous gland adenomas are benign epithelial neoplasms of the lung. Previous nomenclature includes adenomatous polyps of the bronchus, bronchial cystadenomas, bronchial adenomas of the mucous gland type, mucous cell adenomas, and papillary cystadenomas. They occur sporadically, affecting men more than women.

Among reported cases, most patients presented with coughing, shortness of breath, and wheezing. Most mucous gland adenomas occur in the mainstem airways and trachea. Although chest radiographs can show a nodular density, or distal atelectasis, imaging studies are often unrevealing. Computed tomography can identify obstructing bronchial lesions, although may underestimate the amount of submucosal invasion. Pathologic examination shows mucus-filled glandular and tubular spaces with an epithelial cell lining. These benign tumors are treated with lung parenchyma sparing resection (ie, bronchial sleeve resection), generally without the need for lobectomy. Those smaller than 3 cm with low mitotic activity are more likely to have a benign course.[12]

Mucinous cystadenoma These are epithelial neoplasms typically found as asymptomatic, peripheral, cystic nodules. Although some are benign, many are malignant or have atypical features. They are often positive for thyroid transcription factor and cytokeratin 7. Because of the high incidence of atypia, complete excision is recommended.

Mesenchymal tumors

Hamartoma The term hamartoma was first applied to benign tumors in the lung composed of fat and cartilage by Goldsworthy in 1934.[13] Lung hamartomas are the most common benign lung tumor, most commonly discovered as asymptomatic radiographic findings.

Hamartomas are generally non-neoplastic, disordered collections of benign tissue normally present in a given organ. In the lung, however, pulmonary hamartomas are benign neoplasms composed of at least two types of mesenchymal tissue. They are typically found in the periphery, although endobronchial hamartomas are occasionally seen (<10%).[14] Chest radiographs classically show a "popcorn" pattern of calcification in 30% of cases. On histopathology, they are often lobulated, and contain a mixture of cartilage, fat, myxoid connective tissue, smooth muscle, or epithelium. The presence of only one type of mesenchymal tissue suggests lipoma, leiomyoma, or chondroma. Cytogenetic abnormalities have been identified in pulmonary hamartomas. Pulmonary hamartomas can be managed either nonoperatively with serial imaging or with wedge resection.

Solitary fibrous tumor of the lung These are typically pleural-based tumors containing bland spindled cells with ingrowths of epithelial cells. Vimentin and CD34 histopathology markers confirm the diagnosis of solitary fibrous tumor. Importantly, solitary fibrous tumors can be mistaken for mesothelioma if thorough immunohistochemistry panels are not used. Although 80% are benign, there is some malignant potential, and resection is generally recommended.[15]

Clear cell (sugar tumor) Clear cell tumors of the lung are rare asymptomatic nodules. Histologically, they are uniform proliferations of clear and granular cells. They must be distinguished from metastastic renal cell carcinoma. Unlike renal cell carcinoma, clear cell tumors of the lung are cytokeratin negative, vimentin negative, and HMB-45 positive. They are not mitotically active, and are generally benign.

Other mesenchymal tumors Nerve Sheath Tumors—rare intrapulmonary tumors histologically similar to schwannomas of other sites. Nerve sheath tumors are often associated with the dorsal root ganglia of spinal nerves and may present with posterior pleural or mediastinal mass.

Leiomyomas—smooth muscle tumors that can be endobronchial or parenchymal

Chrondromas—cartilaginous tumors without epithelial elements

Lipomas—composed of adipose tissue, they are more commonly endobronchial in location, but can be parenchymal

INFECTIOUS AND RHEUMATOLOGIC DISEASE

Pneumonia

Pneumonia is the fifth leading cause of death in the United States among adults 65 years of age and older. Physiologic changes that occur with aging predispose to the development of pneumonia, including impaired mucociliary clearance, increased risk of aspiration because of diminished swallowing reflexes, increased rigidity of the chest wall, and atrophy of respiratory muscles and chronic obstructive airway disease. Elderly patients with pneumonia often present with nonspecific or atypical symptoms such as failure to thrive, confusion, frequent falling, and decreased ability to perform usual daily activities, particularly if they have some level of underlying dementia. The most commonly reported symptom in one study of patients older than 65 with community-acquired pneumonia was dyspnea, followed by cough and fever.[1]

Community-acquired pneumonia remains a substantial cause of morbidity, with about 915,000 cases in the elderly population each year. *Streptococcus pneumoniae* is thought to be the leading cause. Among adults aged 50 or older, there are 24,000 cases of invasive pneumococcal disease (defined by isolation of *Streptococcus pneumoniae* from a normally sterile site, eg, blood or cerebrosprinal fluid), resulting in 4500 deaths.[16]

Increasing age confers greater risk of invasive pneumococcal disease. Compared with adults aged 65 to 74, adults 85 or older have three times the risk of invasive disease. Although the pneumococcal polysaccharide vaccine (PPV) has been shown effective in reducing the risk of invasive pneumococcal disease in immunocompetent older adults, its efficacy at preventing nonbacteremic pneumococcal pneumonia has not been firmly established, nor has its efficacy in preventing invasive pneumococcal disease in immunocompromised older adults. Currently, the Advisory Committee on Immunization Practices recommends that all adults receive a dose of PPV on or after age 65.

The introduction of a conjugate vaccine for young children targeting seven pneumococcal serotypes has resulted in a decreased incidence of pneumococcal disease in older adults. Among adults aged 50 and older, the incidence of disease caused by the seven conjugate vaccine serotypes decreased by 55% in the period after introduction of the vaccine for children. This is thought to be a result of decreased pneumococcal carriage and transmission by young children.[17]

As the epidemiology of community-acquired pneumonia changes, particularly since the advent of the pneumococcal conjugate vaccine in children, so does the potential benefit of the PPV in older adults. From 1998 to 1999, there were 51.7 cases of invasive pneumococcal disease attributable to the 23 serotypes in the PPV per 100,000 older adults; in 2004, there were 26.9 cases per 100,000 older adults.

Empyema

Thoracic infections can be complicated by the development of pleural empyemas: loculated fibrinopurulent collections in the pleural space. Empyemas carry considerable morbidity, and are associated with mortality of up to 20%. Most empyemas result from parapneumonic effusions in patients with pneumonia, with nearly half resulting from infection with gram-positive bacteria (**Table 2**). If untreated, these effusions progress from freely flowing exudates to multiloculated collections. Empyema can result in sepsis, respiratory compromise, and trapped lung.[18]

Thoracic empyema affects roughly 65,000 people annually. A retrospective study of 132 patients in Taiwan compared community-acquired empyema in patients younger than 65 years with those older than 65. Risk factors for the development of empyema in older patients included chronic lung disease, central nervous system disease, malignancy, and diabetes mellitus. Most thoracic empyemas develop as a complication of bronchopulmonary infection, but they can also result from intra-abdominal infection, esophageal fistula, chest trauma, retropharyngeal or periodontal abscesses, and mycotic aortic aneurysms. Older patients were less likely to present with high fevers and chest pain, but more likely to have dyspnea. Microbiology data did not differ significantly from the younger group of patients. Although the older group had increased incidence of respiratory failure, renal failure, shock, and longer hospital stays, the overall mortality was the same. Although earlier surgical intervention led to faster recovery in the younger group of patients, early intervention did not alter the recovery course for older patients.[19]

Given the high incidence of pneumonia in the elderly population, older patients are at an attendant increased risk of developing empyemas. Those elderly patients who reside in nursing homes are at particular risk of developing empyemas following aspiration pneumonia, and presenting with more indolent, subtle symptoms.

A comparison of community-acquired versus nursing home–acquired empyemas found that community-dwelling patients typically presented with dyspnea, fever, and cough, whereas nursing home residents were more likely to present with dyspnea and weight loss. More nursing home residents had multiloculated effusions on computed tomography. Not surprisingly, the success rate of nonsurgical intervention was significantly lower for the nursing home patients.

Anaerobic bacteria were more frequently isolated from the pleural cultures of nursing home residents compared with community dwellers, suggesting that swallowing abnormalities, as one might develop from dementia or cerebrovascular accident, put the patient at high risk of aspiration pneumonia and subsequent empyema

Table 2
Bacterial isolates in empyema in patients aged 65 or older, excluding mycobacterium, both community and nursing home acquired

	Percentage of Positive Pleural Cultures	
Organism	**Tsai et al[19]**	**El Solh et al[18]**
Aerobic gram-positive	46%	49%
Streptococcus milleri *Viridans streptococci* *Staphylococcus aureus* *Streptococcus pneumoniae*		
Aerobic gram-negative	24%	27%
Escherichia coli *Klebsiella pneumoniae* *Proteus mirabilis* *Pseudomonas aeruginosa*		
Anaerobic	21%	26%
Peptostreptococcus species *Bacteroides* species *Prevotella* species *Fusobacterium* species		
Fungal	9%	
Candida albicans *Nonalbicans Candida*		

development. Oral and dental hygiene thus remains a potentially modifiable risk factor in the elderly nursing home patient population. Speech and language specialists can be indispensable in detecting patients at high risk for aspiration.

Elderly patients undergoing thoracoscopic or open evacuation of empyema and pneumolysis have higher mortality rates than younger patients. One study found surgery-related mortality rates of 3.46% in patients younger than 70, versus 18.3% in patients older than 70 years undergoing surgical treatment of thoracic empyema. Risk factors for surgery-related mortality in the elderly population included the presence of lung abscess, necrotizing pneumonitis, and preoperative ventilatory dependency. This is perhaps related to decreased physiologic reserve, with respiratory muscle atrophy, and resultant reduced force-generating capacity of the respiratory muscles.[20]

Rheumatoid Pleural Effusions

Although rare, pleural effusions can develop as a complication of rheumatoid arthritis (RA). Although clinically significant effusions are uncommon, pleural involvement is the most frequent manifestation of RA in the chest, and pleural effusions can be the initial presentation of previously undiagnosed RA. Men with high rheumatoid factor titers are most likely to be affected.

Rheumatoid pleural effusions result from rheumatoid nodules on the parietal pleural surface, increasing the permeability of pleural capillaries and decreasing egress of fluid from the pleural cavity. These nodules are occasionally seen during thoracoscopic biopsies as numerous small vesicles or granules, giving the parietal pleura a "gritty" appearance. Mesothelial cells are replaced by a pseudo-stratified epithelioid cell layer that is easily detached, leaving an inflamed pleural surface with impaired pleural fluid absorption. Rheumatoid pleural effusions are exudative, with lymphocytic predominance. Tadpole cells (likely of macrophage origin), palisades of epithelioid cells, and a lack of mesothelial cells in the pleural fluid are suggestive of rheumatoid effusion.

Most rheumatoid pleural effusions resolve in an average of 14 months, and they are typically treated with repeated aspiration if clinically indicated. However, some patients will require pleurectomy for nonexpanding lung. Pleural biopsy is indicated only in atypical cases of rheumatoid pleural effusion—those patients without arthritis, with a chylous effusion, or when tuberculosis or malignancy is suspected. Ruling out infection and malignancy are critical, particularly because therapy for RA involves immunosuppressive agents as well as new biologic therapies.[21,22]

SUMMARY

The spectrum of benign thoracic disease in the elderly includes structural abnormalities, infectious disease and their complications, benign neoplastic growths, and autoimmune disease. Differences in physiologic reserve in this population make diagnosis difficult, as elderly patients may not present in the classic fashion, as well as complicate treatment. Benign thoracic disease in the elderly can pose a challenging clinical problem. Older patients with comorbid diseases may have poor tolerance of unnecessary surgical interventions. However, benign disorders of the chest associated with symptoms attributable to effusion or obstruction of airways can limit quality of life. Minimally invasive techniques (eg, video-assisted thoracoscopic surgery) can limit the morbidity associated with intervention. Additionally, prompt intervention may spare the patient more invasive treatments. For example, early effusions can be managed with simple drainage rather than thoracotomy and decortication.

With respect to suspected benign thoracic lesions in the elderly, guiding principles for management include avoiding unnecessary interventions while not overlooking potential malignancies. Close surveillance of progressive symptoms, ensuring no radiographic change in the size of the lesion over 2 years, and use of positron-emission tomography remain the diagnostic keys to accurate management.

REFERENCES

1. Torres M, Moayedi S. Evaluation of the acutely dyspneic elderly patient. Clin Geriatr Med 2007;23: 307–25.
2. Pereira de Godoy JM, Godoy MF, Batigalia F, et al. The association of Mondor's disease with protein S deficiency: case report and review of literature. J Thromb Thrombolysis 2002;13(3):187–9.
3. Sulaiman A, Cottin V, De Souza Neto EP, et al. Cough-induced intercostals lung herniation requiring surgery: report of a case. Surg Today 2006;36:978–80.
4. Athanassiadi K, Bagaev E, Simon A, et al. Lung herniation: a rare complication in minimally invasive cardiothoracic surgery. Eur J Cardiothorac Surg 2008;33:774–6.
5. Caceres M, Ali SZ, Braud R, et al. Spontaneous pneumomediastinum: a comparative study and review of the literature. Ann Thorac Surg 2008;86: 962–6.
6. De Bari M, Chiarlone M, Matteuzzi D, et al. Thoracic kyphosis and ventilatory dysfunction in unselected older persons: an epidemiological study in Dicomano, Italy. J Am Geriatr Soc 2004;52:909–15.
7. Harrison RA, Siminoski K, Vethanayagam D, et al. Osteoporosis-related kyphosis and impairments in pulmonary function: a systematic review. J Bone Miner Res 2007;22(3):447–57.
8. Yang HL, Zhao L, Liu J, et al. Changes of pulmonary function for patients with osteoporotic vertebral compression fractures after kyphoplasty. J Spinal Disord Tech 2007;20:221–5.
9. Borczuk AC. Benign tumors and tumorlike conditions of the lung. Arch Pathol Lab Med 2008;132: 1133–48.
10. Beasley MB, Brambilla E, Travis WD. The 2004 World Health Organization classification of lung tumors. Semin Roentgenol 2005;40:90–7.
11. Ruan SY, Chen KY, Yang PC. Recurrent respiratory papillomatosis with pulmonary involvement: a case report and review of the literature. Respirology 2009;14:137–40.
12. Milenković B, Stojsić J, Mandarić D, et al. Mucous gland adenoma simulating bronchial asthma: case report and literature review. J Asthma 2007;44: 789–93.
13. Goldsworthy NE. Chondroma of the lung (Hamartoma chondromatosum pulmonis). J Pathol Bacteriol 1934; 39(2):291–8.
14. Cosio BG, Villena V, Echave-Sustaeta J, et al. Endobronchial hamartoma. Chest 2002;122:202–5.
15. Jenkins LA, O-Yurvati AH. Solitary fibrous pleural tumor. J Am Osteopath Assoc 2008;108(6):307–9.
16. Jackson LA, Janoff EN. Pneumococcal vaccination of elderly adults: new paradigms for protection. Vaccine 2008;47:1328–38.
17. Lexau CA, Lynfield R, Danila R, et al. Changing epidemiology of invasive pneumococcal disease among older adults in the era of pediatric pneumococcal conjugate vaccine. J Am Med Assoc 2005; 294(16):2043–51.
18. El Solh AA, Alhajjhasan A, Ramadan F, et al. A comparative study of community- and nursing home-acquired empyema thoracis. J Am Geriatr Soc 2007;55(11):1847–52.
19. Tsai TH, Jerng JS, Chen KY, et al. Community-acquired thoracic empyema in older people. J Am Geriatr Soc 2005;53:1203–9.
20. Hsieh MJ, Liu YH, Chao YK, et al. Risk factors in surgical management of thoracic empyema in elderly patients. ANZ J Surg 2008;78:445–8.
21. Balbir-Gurman A, Yigla M, Nahir AM, et al. Rheumatoid pleural effusion. Semin Arthritis Rheum 2006;35: 368–78.
22. Avnon LS, Aby-Shakra M, Flusser D, et al. Pleural effusion associated with rheumatoid arthritis: what cell predominance to anticipate? Rheumatol Int 2007;27:919–25.

Benign Esophageal Disease in the Elderly

M. Blair Marshall, MD, FACS

KEYWORDS

- Benign esophageal disease • Primary motor disorders
- Pharyngeal disorders • Esophageal disease in the elderly
- Diagnosis esophageal disorders
- Treatment esophageal disorders

The diagnosis and management of benign esophageal disease in the elderly based on age alone should not necessarily be different from that in the general population; however, the comorbidities associated with an aging population are critical factors that impact the morbidity and mortality associated with treating this population, predominantly in the surgical management of benign esophageal disease. With improvements in diagnostic tools, anesthesia and pain management, as well as overall perioperative care, the morbidity and mortality of surgical interventions for the management of benign esophageal disease have decreased over the past decades.

The treatment of benign disease of the esophagus should be determined by the symptoms and their affect on quality of life. Any plan for intervention must take into consideration the patient's comorbidities, life expectancy, and quality of life. Once this is determined, the therapeutic options to improve these symptoms may be considered in the context of the relative risks of various interventions, life expectancy, and subsequent quality of life with each therapeutic option.

Currently, most symptomatic benign esophageal pathologies can be managed with a variety of minimally invasive techniques, decreasing the morbidity of these procedures and minimizing the need for significant recovery periods or prolonged hospital stays. For emergent procedures, the postoperative morbidity and mortality remain significant despite an improvement in outcomes.[1] Nevertheless, technologic advances have allowed one to take a selective approach in the management of these patients, minimizing the morbidity and mortality in some settings. Literature on this subject, specific for the elderly, is scant and must be extrapolated from larger patient series that are not limited solely to the management of elderly patients. The care of the patient with a primary motor disorder of the esophagus is complex. There is a lack of universal agreement on the diagnostic criteria for many of these disorders as well as a lack of consensus on optimal therapy. Multiple options for treatment are presented for most of these disorders, although with a less invasive treatment option, usually there is a corresponding lower rate of success associated with its use.

This article discusses the diagnosis and management of benign esophageal disease in the elderly, including motility disorders, leiomyoma, duplication cysts, strictures, diverticula, and perforation. Barrett's esophagus in the context of reflux disease is reviewed but not its management as a premalignant condition (as this is adressed in another chapter). Because the current definition of elderly is a patient aged more than 65 years, this article represents a spectrum of therapeutic options depending not only age but also on associated comorbidities and life expectancy. Clinical judgment dictates that all elderly patients undergoing a surgical procedure should have a preoperative cardiopulmonary evaluation, and these results should be weighed when planning any intervention. Pulmonary function testing should be performed; a forced expiratory volume in 1 second (FEV_1) of less than 1.25 L is a relative contraindication to any major operation.

Division of Thoracic Surgery, Georgetown University Medical Center, Georgetown University School of Medicine, 4 PHC, 3800 Reservoir Road, NW, Washington, DC 20007, USA
E-mail address: mbm5@gunet.georgetown.edu

Thorac Surg Clin 19 (2009) 321–332
doi:10.1016/j.thorsurg.2009.07.002
1547-4127/09/$ – see front matter

thoracic.theclinics.com

PRIMARY AND SECONDARY MOTOR DYSFUNCTION OF THE ESOPHAGUS

Diagnosis and Management of Pharyngeal Esophageal Disorders

Acquired pharyngoesophageal swallowing disorders demonstrate increased frequency in the elderly because they are associated with other comorbidities that increase with age such as cerebral vascular accidents. As the cerebral cortex and brainstem combine to control the oral phase of swallowing, central nervous system dysfunction can result in dysphagia at the oral pharyngeal level. Disorders of the pharyngoesophageal phase of swallowing result in dysphagia, pharyngeal regurgitation, and aspiration. Defective mechanisms involved in pathology at this level include inadequate oropharyngeal bolus transport, an inability to pressurize the pharynx, an inability to elevate the larynx, incoordination of cricopharyngeal relaxation and pharyngeal contraction, and decreased compliance of the pharynx and proximal esophagus.[2]

Evaluation of the patient complaining of oral pharyngeal dysphagia includes several studies. Clinical assessment should give rise to the underlying pathology leading to oral pharyngeal dysfunction; these entities may include cerebral infarcts, cervical spine disorders, amyotrophic lateral sclerosis, Parkinson's disease, brainstem tumors, poliomyositis, pseudobulbar palsy, peripheral neuropathy, or damage to the cranial nerves involved in swallowing. Muscular diseases including dermatomyositis, myotonic dystrophy, and myasthenia gravis are less common.

Video- or cineradiography is the most useful test to evaluate the oropharyngeal bolus and conditions of deglutition, bolus propulsion, and transit. Aberrancies such as swallowing hesitation, pharyngeal stasis, functional obstruction, upper esophageal sphincter dysfunction, epiglottic dysfunction, and tracheal aspiration can be demonstrated. In addition, when performed concurrently with manometry, the anatomic and functional abnormalities may be simultaneously addressed, giving a more comprehensive view of the underlying disorder and options for management.

Due to the spacing of the side ports, traditional manometric probes are inadequate for evaluation of esophagopharyngeal dysfunction; therefore, one must use either the Dent sleeve technique or a specialized catheter in which the side ports are 1 cm apart for a distance of 8 cm. With this technique, one is able to record pharyngeal resting pressures, contraction pressures, and their duration to evaluate the pharyngoesophageal junction.[3]

A complete and thorough evaluation leads to the development of an effective strategy for treatment, including rehabilitation techniques, cricopharyngeal myotomy, botulism toxin injections, or dilation when appropriate. The underlying pathophysiology leading to dysphagia dictates the therapeutic options. Because stroke patients may continue to improve further out from the event, any consideration of surgical intervention should be postponed for at least 6 months following an event. These techniques are aimed at improving the patient's quality of life while minimizing the complications associated with orpharyngeal dysphagia.[4] Currently, controversy exists in regard to the optimal management strategy because there are few studies that identify the correct indications, complications of intervention, and outcomes associated with these strategies.

In select patients, cricopharyngeal myotomy may be performed and has demonstrated improvement in dysphagia; however, because these patients tend to have significant comorbidities, the procedure is not without risk of morbidity and mortality. In particular, the development of pulmonary complications postoperatively is associated with a high mortality.[5] In those patients considered too high risk for cricopharyngeal myotomy, paralysis of the sphincter with botulism toxin may alleviate symptoms in approximately 40%; however, despite this being a fairly minimal procedure, complications are significant owing to the underlying high-risk candidates in whom this procedure is performed.[6]

Diagnosis and Management of Motor Disorders of the Body of the Esophagus

The underlying cause of primary esophageal motor disorders is not known. Without a full understanding of the pathophysiology of these disorders, there is lack of consensus on the diagnostic criteria as well as optimal treatment strategy. Primary motor abnormalities of the esophagus center on abnormalities of the muscular coordination of the esophageal body or the muscular function of the lower esophageal sphincter (LES) or a combination of both. Dysfunction of these structures can give rise to a variety of symptoms, including chest pain, odynophagia, dysphagia, weight loss, reflux, and aspiration. Primary esophageal motor disorders are best classified into six subtypes as defined by Spechler and Castell:[7] classic achalasia, atypical disorders of LES relaxation, diffuse esophageal spasm, isolated hypertensive LES, and ineffective esophageal motility (IEM). The latter was previously labeled as nonspecific esophageal motility disorder. Evaluation of the underlying problem leading to symptoms includes a variety of diagnostic tests. Appropriate tests for the evaluation of underlying pathophysiology of esophageal motor disorders include radiographic imaging, esophagoscopy, manometry, 24-hour pH testing, esophageal scintigraphy, acid clearing tests, and various provocative tests.[8] These tests are well tolerated even in patients with multiple comorbidities. Secondary motor disorders of the esophagus include collagen vascular disease, neuromuscular disease, infection, endocrine disorders, metastatic disease, and idiopathic pseudo-obstruction. Management of these disorders is akin to management of the underlying disease process; therefore, they are not discussed herein.

Videofluoroscopy

Videofluoroscopy is the initial diagnostic maneuver for determining the underlying pathophysiology in patients presenting with dysphagia.[9] It is useful for the exclusion of underlying neoplasm and gives clues toward the diagnosis. Video recording or barium swallows allow for slow motion evaluation of the swallowing mechanism. At least five wet swallows are performed and recorded. In achalasia, the typical bird's beak pattern at the gastroesophageal junction is usually seen (**Fig. 1**). In addition, proximal dilation of the esophagus will give additional clues on the function of the body of the esophagus. In diffuse esophageal spasm, repetitive nonperistaltic contractions cause the typical "corkscrew" appearance on a barium esophagram; however, the radiographic findings in all of these disorders, including achalasia, diffuse esophageal spasm, nutcracker esophagus, hypertensive LES, or IEM, may be minimal, nonspecific, or pronounced. The interpretation of these findings with the additional information obtained from other studies puts the pathology into context. In the diagnosis and management of gastroesophageal reflux disease (GERD), radiographic assessment evaluates anatomic abnormalities such as the presence of a hiatal hernia, shortened esophagus, erosive esophagitis, or stricture.

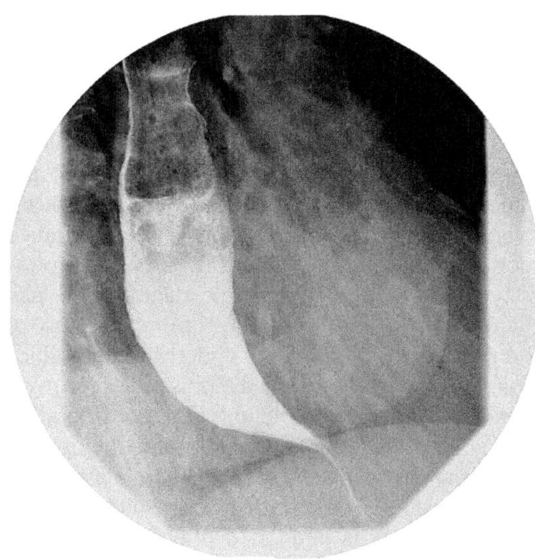

Fig. 1. Radiographic image of a patient with achalasia. Note the typical bird's beak pattern at the LES.

Manometry

Esophageal manometry remains the gold standard for evaluation of the motor function of the esophagus. It is performed by using several capillary catheters that are perfused with water. The catheters have radial side ports of varying distances along their length. This low compliance pneumohydraulic system has an infusion rate of 0.6 mL/min. The catheter is connected to external transducers and then passed through the nose and into the stomach. Pressures are recorded as the catheter is slowly withdrawn across the LES into the body of the esophagus. A rise in pressure from the baseline gastric reading identifies the LES. The respiratory inversion point (RIP) occurs when the positive-pressure reading associated with breathing becomes negative, suggesting that this portion of the catheter is now intrathoracic. By measuring the distance between the LES to the RIP, one can calculate the length of the intra-abdominal LES.

Withdrawal of the catheter across the sphincter is usually performed manually or through a continuous automated technique. For the evaluation of relaxation of the LES, the probe is placed so that the side holes are positioned within the stomach, at the high pressure zone and within the body of the esophagus. Five to ten wet swallows are performed while pressure tracings are recorded. During the swallow, when the LES relaxes, the sphincter pressure should drop to that of the stomach.

To evaluate the body of the esophagus, the catheter is positioned so that all of the side holes are within the body of the esophagus. To standardize this part, the most proximal side hole is positioned 1 cm below the level of the upper esophageal sphincter. Ten wet swallows are performed and the pressure tracings recorded.

Because of the intermittent nature of motor abnormalities, standard manometry in a laboratory has limitations. Prolonged pressure recordings performed over a 24-hour period have allowed for a more accurate portrayal of esophageal motility. This method may be particularly important for the evaluation of GERD, which may be sporadic in nature.

Twenty-four hour pH monitoring

Given that many patients with chronic reflux disease may be relatively asymptomatic, the definition of reflux disease should rely on 24-hour pH monitoring. The test is performed by placing a small pH electrode passed through the nose into the esophagus with the distal tip lying 5 cm above the upper border of the LES. Intraluminal pH is measure continuously every 4 seconds over a 24-hour period, and the data are recorded on a portable data manager. All medications interfering with gastrointestinal activity are stopped to prevent their interference with the results. During the test the patient is instructed on maintaining a detailed diary of their oral intake and activities. Esophageal exposure is best measured as the cumulative time that the pH is below a specific threshold, usually 4, the frequency of reflux episodes, the duration of episodes, and the longest episode. The test is used not only to demonstrate the presence of GERD but also to predict the likelihood and severity of mucosal injury related to chronic reflux disease. Although increasing age is associated with an increased exposure of the esophagus to acid, the severity of symptoms of reflux decreases with increased age.[10]

Endoscopy

Upper endoscopy is essential in any patient undergoing evaluation of esophageal dysmotility for the exclusion of underlying organic pathology. In this setting, a careful retroflexed view from the gastric side of the gastroesophageal junction is necessary to exclude malignancy. In the evaluation of GERD, 24-hour pH monitoring has replaced esophagoscopy as the gold standard for diagnosis because only two thirds of patient with reflux have esophagitis at endoscopy.[11] Biopsies should be done at the time of endoscopy and may increase the sensitivity of the diagnosis of esophagitis. Biopsies and brushings should be performed on all strictures to exclude malignancy and are required to diagnose Barrett's esophagus. Flames of reddish mucosa can be viewed extending proximal from the gastroesophageal junction. In this setting, multiple biopsies are necessary to detect high-grade dysplasia or carcinoma in situ, which may be present without any visual clues. For accurate mapping, biopsy specimens are taken at each quadrant, every centimeter along the entire length of metaplastic mucosa.

MANAGEMENT OF PRIMARY ESOPHAGEAL MOTOR DISORDERS

Achalasia

Achalasia is the most common of the primary motor disorders of the esophagus and affects as many as 6 in 100,000 persons. It is a heterogeneous disease and presents with a variety of findings. All patients presenting with dysphagia should undergo videofluoroscopy, endoscopy, manometry, and pH monitoring. Although many functional abnormalities of the esophagus can be observed in patients with achalasia, the primary dysfunction is failure of the LES to relax (**Fig. 2**). This failure results in pooling of swallowed material in the distal esophagus, leading to reflux and aspiration. The esophagus proximal to the sphincter may demonstrate aperistalsis or simultaneous repetitive contractions, such as that seen in diffuse esophageal spasm. Therapeutic options for the management of symptomatic achalasia range from medications to surgical intervention. In the management of symptomatic achalasia in the elderly, durability of the repair may be less of a concern than minimizing periprocedural morbidity and mortality. Certainly, considerations for management in a 65-year-old patient may be quite different from that in an 85-year-old patient, although in the latter, associated comorbidities will likely have a larger role. The majority of data suggest that long-term durability and quality of life are best achieved with a laparoscopic myotomy and partial fundoplication, and in younger patients this is the recommended treatment. Because this operation is more invasive than pneumatic dilation, the relative risks must be considered because the comorbidities increase for each particular patient. There are no randomized prospective studies comparing these interventions in this population. Through a recursive decision-tree analysis, Heller myotomy is associated with the longest quality-adjusted survival. Pneumatic dilation therapy is favored when the effectiveness of laparoscopic surgery at relieving dysphagia is less than 89.7%, the operative mortality risk is greater than 0.7%, or the probability of reflux after pneumatic dilatation is less than 19%.[12,13] In this setting, the relative risk of the procedure, the patients underlying comorbidities, and the relative local expertise in performing these procedures are taken into consideration when determining the optimal therapeutic option.

Botulism toxin injection is another relatively low-risk procedure. The durability of results with this type of therapy is inferior to pneumatic dilation; however, the relative risk is lower. Consideration of this therapy is again dependent on the patient's

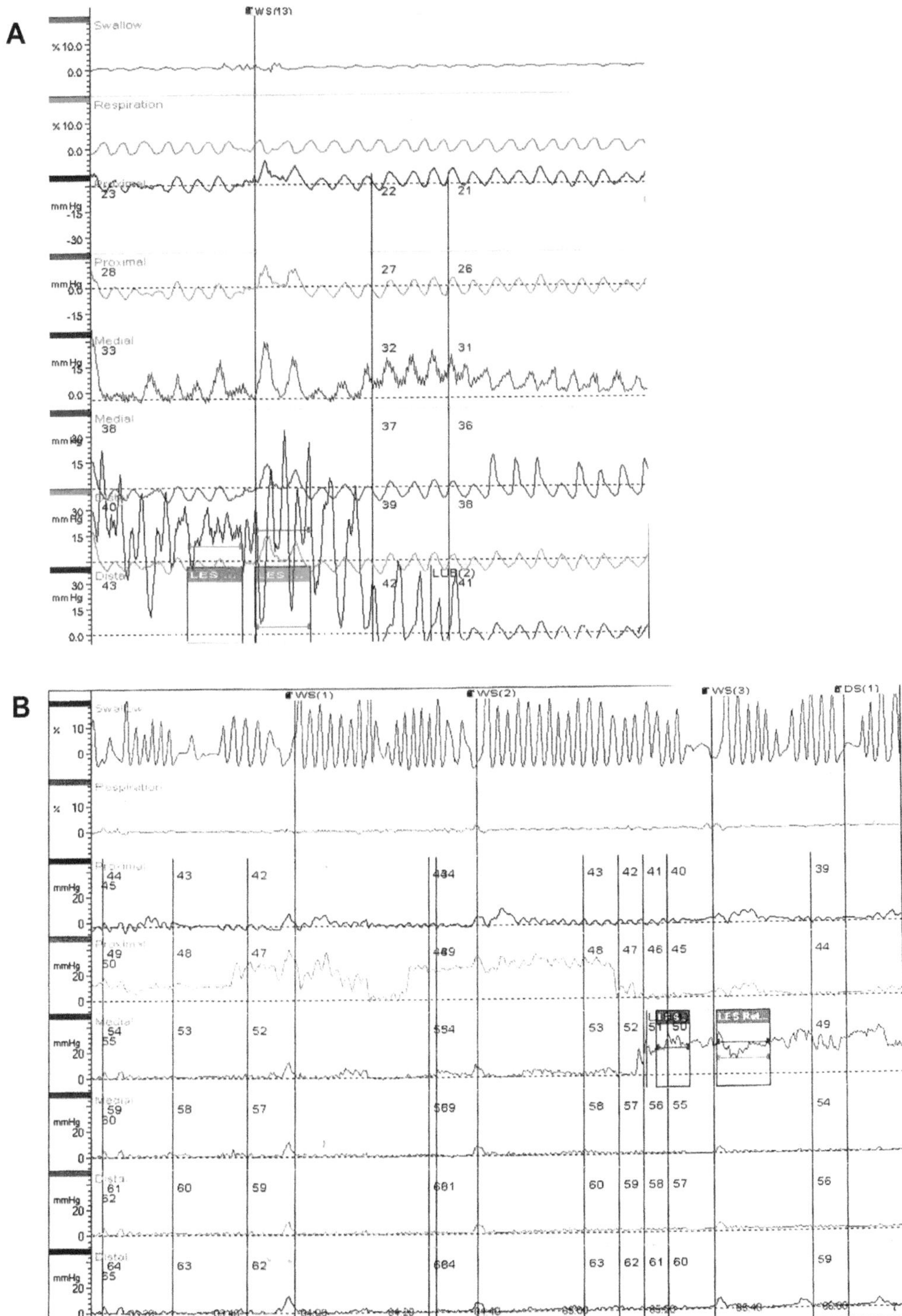

Fig. 2. Manometric tracing in two patients with achalasia. (*A*) Tracing demonstrates increased pressure at the LES. (*B*) Tracing demonstrates increase LES pressure with aperistalsis of the esophageal body.

comorbidities and the relative risk of other more durable procedures. One series reported on the use of botulism toxin for symptomatic elderly patients with American Society of Anesthesiologists class III or IV disease. In this small series, 16 of 20 patients had symptomatic relief.[14] Of the patients who failed initial treatment, three of four went on to have an uneventful balloon dilation. The remaining patients underwent percutaneous gastrostomy tube placement.

Medical therapy such as nifedipine may be tried, although objective data on the effectiveness of this treatment strategy are scarce. Nifedipine has been demonstrated to decrease LES sphincter pressure by 28%; however, most agree that it should not be considered as an alternative to dilation or myotomy. The demonstrated change in sphincter pressure is not necessarily associated with an improvement in symptoms. Because there is minimal morbidity associated with this treatment strategy and it may improve quality of life in a select few, it may be an option in patients whose comorbidities prevent the use of more invasive strategies.[15]

For patients who have already undergone a myotomy or potentially a repeat myotomy who again develop symptoms, esophagectomy may be the only remaining option. Select patients, even the elderly, can do well with this operation (**Fig. 3**). When performed in patients with normal esophageal motor function, this operation may not be well tolerated as far as postoperative quality of life; however, when performed in patients with dysphagia and achalasia, the improvement in quality of life, even in the elderly, can be remarkable.[16]

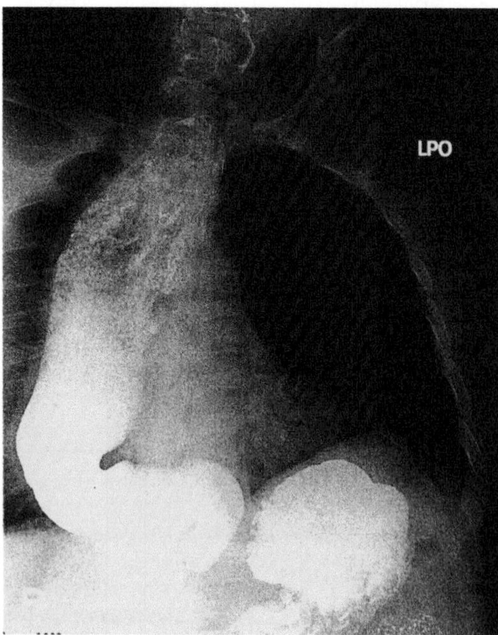

Fig. 3. Barium esophagram showing changes associated with end-stage achalasia, a dilated sigmoid esophagus in an elderly patient. This patient initially did well following thoracotomy and myotomy. Ten years later, symptoms recurred and he underwent laparoscopic repeat myotomy. Six years following this procedure, the patient underwent an uneventful esophagectomy.

Diffuse Esophageal Spasm

Patients with diffuse esophageal spasm present clinically with complaints of dysphagia and chest pain. Radiographic studies demonstrate tertiary contractions and repetitive simultaneous contractions of the muscular body of the esophagus. These contractions are frequently of high amplitude or prolonged duration followed by a period of intermittent normal peristalsis. Although this disorder can affect the entire length of the esophagus, it is most commonly limited to the distal two thirds of the body of the esophagus. The diagnostic hallmark of this disorder is the simultaneous nonperistaltic contractions in the smooth muscle of the esophagus in at least 20% of wet swallows, although this would be debated by some.[17]

Before considering any intervention, a complete evaluation of the foregut should be performed because there is a high rate of other associated disorders that should be taken into consideration when planning treatment options. Medical therapy aimed at relaxing the smooth muscle of the esophagus can be tried. These agents include nitrates, calcium channel blockers, and antimuscarinic agents. Nitroglycerin has shown some symptomatic improvement in patients with diffuse esophageal spasm.[18] Injection of botulism toxin into the muscular fibers of the distal esophagus has demonstrated some benefit but is associated with the necessary repeated injections.[19,20]

In the elderly patient who fails lesser more conservative therapies, thoracoscopic or laparoscopic myotomy may be well tolerated and resolve symptoms. Because the procedure abolishes the high amplitude contractions as well as the peristaltic waves, the myotomy must be extended onto the LES. Dysphagia improves when the benefit of abolishing the simultaneous contractions exceeds the adverse effect of the loss of peristaltic waves; therefore, there is a precarious balance between the benefit and harm associated with this procedure. Diffuse esophageal spasm is a rare disorder. Because of a lack on consensus regarding its diagnosis, it is difficult to compare studies as the patient populations are variable.

Nutcracker Esophagus

Patients with a nutcracker esophagus complain of dysphagia and chest pain as well; however, manometry demonstrates peristaltic waves in the esophagus with a mean amplitude 2 standard deviations above normal. Again, there is a universal lack of agreement on the diagnostic criteria for nutcracker esophagus, and for patients who are severely symptomatic, treatment strategies parallel that of diffuse esophageal spasm.

Ineffective Esophageal Motility

IEM is demonstrated by peristaltic failure. Manometry demonstrates distal esophageal contractions of very low amplitude, less than 30 mm Hg. It is defined by failure of bolus clearance of the esophagus by fluoroscopy. IEM has been associated with GERD (20%–50%), especially in patients whose symptoms are a result of failure to clear the esophagus of acid. To date, there are no effective therapies for the management of this disorder.

Gastroesophageal Reflux Disease

Most patients with chronic GERD are managed for years with medical therapy. Many of these patients complain of chronic pain and other reflux-related symptoms. Over the past several years there has been a flurry of excitement over new endoscopic strategies for the treatment of reflux disease, including radiofrequency ablation, implantation of foreign bulking agents, and tissue apposition devices. The majority of these strategies have been abandoned due to severe adverse events, lack of efficacy, or lack of adoption.[21] There are few randomized controlled clinical trials governing the introduction of these new techniques. Currently, proton pump inhibitors, although expensive, are the mainstay of treatment. Elderly patients with esophagitis respond well to medical therapy, and continuance of treatment is associated with decreased relapse as the patient continues to age.[22]

For patients who have persistent symptoms, who experience complications on medical therapy, or who are dissatisfied with their treatment, surgical fundoplication has demonstrated good long-term results with minimal risk.[23] A complete evaluation of the esophagus must be performed before selecting the optimal surgical intervention. Radiographic imaging demonstrates the presence of structural abnormalities such as associated hiatal hernia or esophageal shortening. Additional studies include endoscopy, manometery, and 24-hour pH monitoring. Esophageal manometry is able to determine the propulsive force on the esophagus necessary for a bolus of food to transit across a newly tightened valve and can highlight associated motility dysfunction such as IEM. Before performing any intervention, one must carefully evaluate the position of the crus, the location of the squamocolumnar junction, and the presence of mucosal injury or stricture defined by inability to pass a 36F endoscope. Failure to take into consideration associated abnormalities such as these and also including IEM leads to poor results. These issues are important to identify preoperatively and need to be addressed at the time of intervention. Failure to recognize esophageal shortening can lead to increased tension on the repair and subsequent breakdown or recurrence of a hiatal hernia. Once the disease has progressed to include an esophageal motility disorder, esophageal shortening, and Barrett's metaplasia, the results of repair in these patients are worse when associated with such end-stage disease. Nevertheless, even in patients with advanced disease, appropriate surgical management is associated with good long-term results and minimal morbidity and mortality.

DIAGNOSIS AND MANAGEMENT OF ESOPHAGEAL DIVERTICULAR DISEASE

Zenker's Diverticulum

A Zenker's diverticulum is an out pouching of the posterior pharyngeal mucosa through Killian's triangle, defined by the oblique fibers of the cricopharyngeus and the inferior constrictor. Most patients present with dysphagia among other complaints, including regurgitation, pain, coughing, weight loss, halitosis, and aspiration. The majority of diverticuli present on the left side of the neck and can be classified into three stages: stage I, minimal; stage II, clearly visible; and stage III, a large diverticulum. Although the pathophysiology of a Zenker's diverticulum is not entirely worked out, the general consensus is that it results from a discoordination of the cricopharyngeus and esophagus. Complete neurologic evaluation to ensure that there are no associated neurologic defects such as laryngeal nerve dysfunction is a necessary step in the evaluation. Small asymptomatic diverticuli do not necessarily require intervention. Large diverticuli can become symptomatic, necessitating intervention.

Current surgical management is institution dependent. A diverticulectomy with myotomy has historically been associated with significant morbidity and mortality; however, this finding is more a reflection of the patient population than the procedure.[24,25] With recent advances in perioperative management, the morbidity has decreased. The endoscopic stapled approach has demonstrated good results as well. Although the open approach offers more durable long-term results, there is less morbidity associated with the endoscopic approach, justifying its use in the elderly population.[26] The endoscopic technique is a transoral division of the common wall between the diverticulum and esophagus, essentially dividing the cricopharyngeus and obliterating the diverticulum. This procedure is facilitated through use of the Weerda diverticuloscope and tailoring of the distal tip of the endoscopic stapler. Placement of a traction suture on the common wall to bring it into the orifice of the stapler also assists in the subsequent division of this common wall. In patients with diverticuli less than 3 cm, those with inadequate opening of their oral cavity, or those with cervical osteoarthritis in whom the cervical spine cannot be adequately extended, this procedure is contraindicated because one cannot obtain the appropriate angle with the rigid instruments needed to complete the procedure. In this setting, because these diverticuli can be symptomatic, an open approach with diverticulectomy for large diverticuli or diverticulopexy for small diverticuli with myotomy is well tolerated, even in the elderly. Specific data in this select population are lacking.[27] In the past, a conservative approach to postoperative management had been associated with a longer hospital stay. More recently, the diverticulum is stapled at the base, the wound closed, and patients advanced on their diet and sent home on postoperative day 1 or 2.

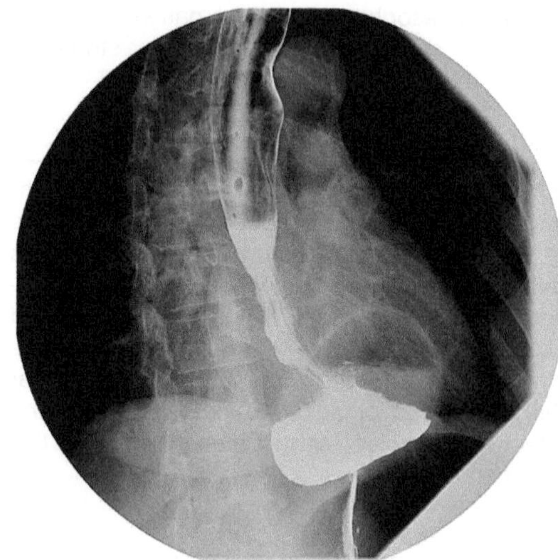

Fig. 4. Barium esophagram demonstrating a large epiphrenic diverticulum.

Epiphrenic Diverticuli

Epiphrenic diverticuli are rare pulsion pseudodiverticuli that are frequently associated with esophageal motility disorders. Because of this, they must be managed within the context that they arise and the underlying pathophysiology corrected, or treatment is associated with a high relapse rate. As is true for other motor disorders, videofluoroscopy, endoscopy, and manometry are critical diagnostics tests (**Fig. 4**). The current mainstay of surgical therapy is a laparoscopic transhiatal excision of the diverticulum with a myotomy and partial fundoplication. Care must be taken during perioperative management to prevent aspiration of diverticular contents that would lead to significant morbidity and mortality in these patients. At the author's center, patients are placed on a liquid diet for 2 days before the procedure. At the time of surgery, they are intubated in the semi-upright position to prevent aspiration. Following endoscopic dissection and resection of the diverticulum, the extent of proximal myotomy on the esophagus is determined by the associated muscular pathology in the body of the esophagus, as determined by preoperative manometric studies. Given the current techniques for accurate diagnosis of the pathophysiology associated with the diverticulum and the newer techniques of minimally invasive surgery, surgical intervention is relatively well tolerated and has a high rate of success in the elderly. For patients considered too high risk to undergo surgical intervention, there are sporadic reports of the successful use of botulism toxin.[28]

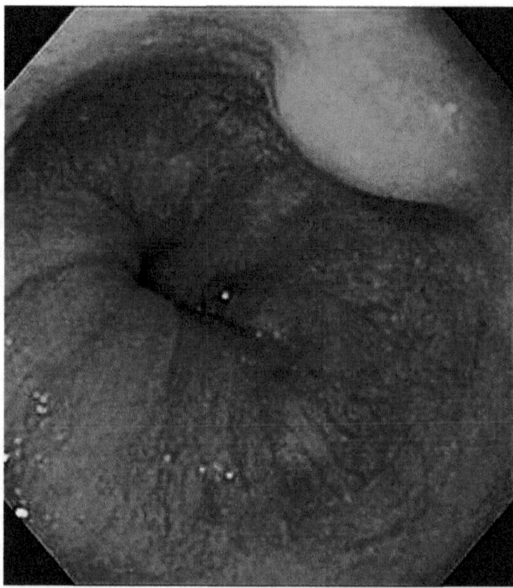

Fig. 5. Endoscopic view of an esophageal leiomyoma protruding into the lumen of the esophagus.

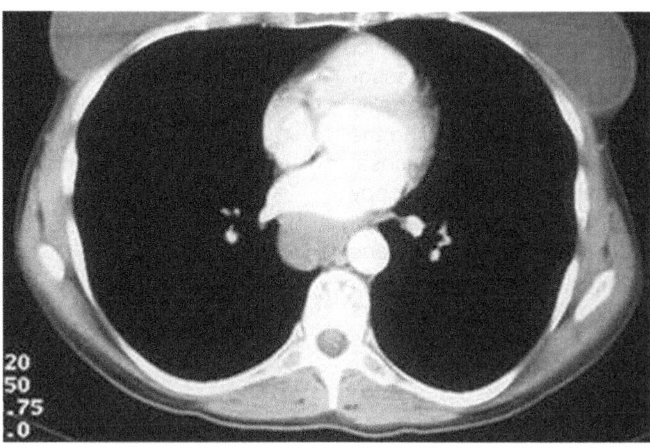

Fig. 6. CT demonstrating an esophageal duplication cyst.

DIAGNOSIS AND MANAGEMENT OF ESOPHAGEAL LEIOMYOMA AND DUPLICATION CYSTS

Leiomyoma and duplication cysts are the most common benign lesions of the esophagus. Current classification of leiomyomas should be along the spectrum of gastrointestinal stromal tumors (GIST). Leiomyomas are five times more common than duplication cysts but are discussed together herein because the diagnosis and management are similar. Approximately one half of patents with leiomyoma and one third of those with esophageal cysts are asymptomatic, and these lesions are usually picked up on evaluation for other problems.

In the evaluation of patients with dysphagia or noncardiac chest pain, barium swallow may reveal a mucosal defect suggestive of a leiomyoma or duplication cyst. Dysphagia is the most common presenting symptom of patients with esophageal leiomyoma. Upper endoscopy usually demonstrates a smooth-walled out pouching of the mucosa into the lumen of the esophagus (**Fig. 5**). This finding usually leads to an endoscopic ultrasound or CT scan for further evaluation of the mass (**Fig. 6**). Endoscopic ultrasound demonstrates a smooth-walled, well-circumscribed tumor, but rarely these lesions can be horseshoe shaped or circumferential as well (**Fig. 7**). The latter types and diffuse esophageal leiomatosis are rare. Endoscopic biopsy demonstrates smooth muscle tumor that stains immunohistochemically negative for c-kit (CD117), CD34, and other markers of a more aggressive GIST.[29]

In elderly patients who are asymptomatic, the lesions can be followed with CT or endoscopic

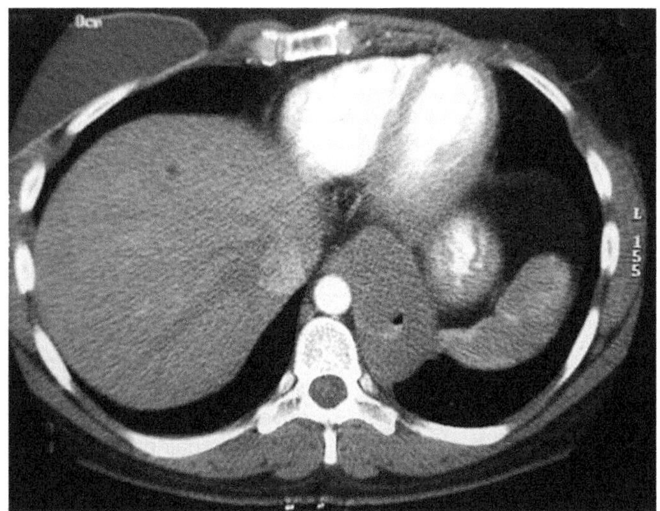

Fig. 7. CT demonstrating a circumferential esophageal leiomyoma.

ultrasound and do not require any intervention. In patients who are significantly symptomatic, video-assisted thoracoscopic enucleation is associated with minimal morbidity and mortality (**Fig. 8**).[30] The mass or cyst is enucleated and the muscle layers reapproximated over the mucosa. The liberal use of intraoperative esophagoscopy to transilluminate the esophageal mucosal wall allows for safe dissection of the submucosal plane between the mucosa and the tumor or cyst (**Fig. 9**). Once the mass is excised, the muscular layers are closed over the mucosa. A barium swallow is obtained the following day, and the patient is discharged home on a soft diet.

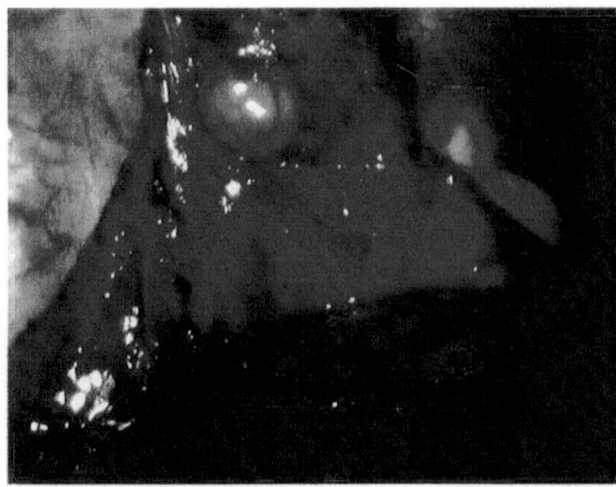

Fig. 9. Transillumination of the esophageal mucosal wall during thoracoscopic resection of a duplication cyst.

BENIGN ESOPHAGEAL STRICTURE AND ESOPHAGEAL WEB

Benign esophageal stricture may result from several causes, including GERD, Schatzki's rings, caustic injury, radiation, or surgical, photodynamic, and sclerotherapy. Many patients present with dysphagia to solids that may eventually progress to liquids. The initial work-up includes a barium esophagram. The evaluation of patients with symptomatic disease should include esophagoscopy with biopsy to rule out malignancy. Therapeutic options for the management of benign esophageal stricture include dilation and high-dose proton pump inhibitors. The majority of patients will respond to this type of therapy. Multiple types of dilation techniques can be used and are successful. Particular techniques should be chosen based on experience and expertise. For patients with refractory strictures, the recent development of self-expanding plastic stents that are relatively easy to remove has become an attractive option for management. Self-expanding metal stents have been previously associated with a high incidence of short- and long-term complications in these patients,[31,32] making the removable plastic stents an attractive option, especially in patients with multiple associated comorbidities. Although the majority of small series reporting on the use of these stents demonstrate a high incidence of complications,[33,34] in patients with multiple comorbidities, this may represent the best therapeutic option.

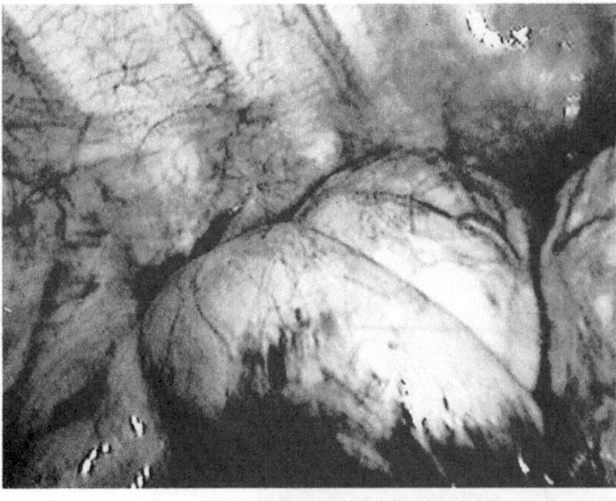

Fig. 8. Thoracoscopic view of esophageal leiomyoma just proximal to the level of the azygous vein.

DIAGNOSIS AND MANAGEMENT OF ESOPHAGEAL PERFORATION

Clinical manifestations of esophageal perforation include severe pain, fever, tachycardia, leukocytosis, and hypotension. A barium esophagram is usually the initial diagnostic test performed, but a CT with oral contrast may give additional information such as the extent of leakage, involvement of pleural space, and soilage. Although the standard approach is surgical intervention including primary repair, aggressive drainage, esophageal resection, or two-stage resection with or without esophagostomy, these procedures can be associated with significant morbidity and mortality in the elderly.[35] More recently, a selective approach to patients presenting with esophageal perforation has been used; the majority of reports are anecdotal. In patients with minimal symptoms and a leukocytosis that is either decreasing or stable, nonoperative management has been described with some success.[36]

Endoscopic closure with clips has been described. There are more reports on the use of covered stents. Stent placement after failed surgical repair or as primary therapy is associated with significant morbidity and a mortality rate of 28%.[37] If the estimated operative morbidity and mortality of a surgical repair are considered excessively high for a particular patient, stent placement should be considered. Other options for high-risk patients include exclusion and diversion with drainage. The initial goal of all of these therapies is to prevent further soilage, sepsis, and death. Gastrointestinal continuity should be considered as a secondary endpoint. As previously discussed, the underlying pathophysiology leading to the perforation must be taken into consideration, as well as each patient's comorbidities before selecting the optimal treatment strategy.

SUMMARY

For the most part, the management of benign esophageal disease in all patients is in evolution. Advances in laparoscopic, thoracoscopic, and endoscopic techniques have lessened the morbidity and mortality associated with the traditional approaches to this pathology. Our understanding of the pathophysiology of primary motor disorders remains incomplete but is certainly more advanced than our understanding just a decade ago. As research continues in this area, our knowledge will increase. Persistent development efforts with industry will continue to provide less invasive options for the management of these patients, and, eventually, the results associated with these techniques will improve as well. For the management of these pathologies in the elderly, the critical issues are the associated comorbidities, the current quality of life, the life expectancy, and the desired quality of life. The optimal treatment strategy may be determined by consideration of all of these factors along with the relative effectiveness and durability of each treatment strategy for the individual elderly patient.

REFERENCES

1. Port JL, Kent MS, Korst RJ, et al. Thoracic esophageal perforations: a decade of experience. Ann. Thorac Surg 2003;75(4):1071–4.
2. Stein HJ, Korn O. Pathophysiology of esophageal motor disorders and gastroesophageal reflux disease. In: Bremner CG, DeMeester T, Peracchia A, editors. Modern approach to benign esophageal disease. St. Louis (MO): Quality Medical Publishing; 1995. p. 1–16.
3. Dire C, Shi G, Manka M, et al. Manometric characteristics of the upper esophageal sphincter recorded with a microsleeve. Am J Gastroenterol 2001;96(5): 1383–9.
4. Cappabianca S, Reginelli A, Monaco L, et al. Combined videofluoroscopy and manometry in the diagnosis of oropharyngeal dysphagia: examination technique and preliminary experience. Radiol Med 2008;113(6):923–40.
5. Brigand C, Ferraro P, Martin J, et al. Risk factors in patients undergoing cricopharyngeal myotomy. Br J Surg 2007;94(8):978–83.
6. Zaninotto G, Marchese Ragona R, Briani C, et al. The role of botulinum toxin injection and upper esophageal sphincter myotomy in treating oropharyngeal dysphagia. J Gastrointest Surg 2004;8(8): 997–1006.
7. Spechler SJ, Castell DO. Classification of oesophageal motility abnormalities. Gut 2001;49(1): 145–51.
8. Constatini M, DeMeester T. Preoperative assessment of esophageal function. In: Bremner CG, DeMeester TR, Peracchia A, editors. Modern approach to benign esophageal pathology. St. Louis (MO): Quality Medical Publishing; 1995. p. 17–56.
9. Schima W, Stacher G, Pokieser P, et al. Esophageal motor disorders: videofluoroscopic and manometric evaluation. Prospective study in 88 symptomatic patients. Radiology 1992;185(2):487–91.
10. Lee J, Anggiansah A, Anggiansah R, et al. Effects of age on the gastroesophageal junction, esophageal motility, and reflux disease. Clin Gastroenterol Hepatol 2007;5(12):1392–8.
11. Fuchs K, DeMeester TR, Albertucci M. Specificity and sensitivity of objective diagnosis of gastroesophageal reflux disease. Surgery 1987;102:575–80.
12. Wang L, Li YM, Li L. Meta-analysis of randomized and controlled treatment trials for achalasia. Dig Dis Sci 2008 [Epub ahead of print].
13. Urbach DR, Hansen PD, Khajanchee YS, et al. A decision analysis of the optimal initial approach to achalasia: laparoscopic Heller myotomy with partial fundoplication, thoracoscopic Heller myotomy, pneumatic dilatation, or botulinum toxin injection. J Gastrointest Surg 2001;5(2):192–205.
14. Wehrmann T, Kokabpick H, Jacobi V, et al. Long-term results of endoscopic injection of botulinum toxin in elderly achalasic patients with tortuous megaesophagus or epiphrenic diverticulum. Endoscopy 1999;31(5):352–8.
15. Bortolotti M. Medical therapy of achalasia: a benefit reserved for few. Digestion 1999;60(1):11–6.
16. Gockel I, Junginger T, Eckardt VF. Persistent and recurrent achalasia after Heller myotomy: analysis of different patterns and long-term results of reoperation. Arch Surg 2007;142(11):1093–7.
17. Almansa C, Hinder RA, Smith CD, et al. A comprehensive appraisal of the surgical treatment of diffuse esophageal spasm. J Gastrointest Surg 2008;12(6): 1133–45.
18. Swamy N. Esophageal spasm: clinical and manometric response to nitroglycerin and long acting nitrites. Gastroenterology 1977;72:23–7.

19. Storr M, Allescher HD, Rosch T, et al. Treatment of symptomatic diffuse esophageal spasm by endoscopic injections of botulinum toxin: a prospective study with long-term follow-up. Gastrointest Endosc. 2001;54:754–9.
20. Patti MG, Pellegrini CA, Arcerito M, et al. Comparison of medical and minimally invasive surgical therapy for primary esophageal motility disorders. Arch Surg 1995;130(6):609–15.
21. Schwartz MP, Wellink H, Gooszen HG, et al. Endoscopic gastroplication for the treatment of gastro-oesophageal reflux disease: a randomised, sham-controlled trial. Gut 2007;56(1):20–8.
22. Pilotto A, Franceschi M, Leandro G, et al. Long-term clinical outcome of elderly patients with reflux esophagitis: a six-month to three-year follow-up study. Am J Ther 2002;9(4):295–300.
23. Grant AM, Wileman SM, Ramsay CR, et al. Minimal access surgery compared with medical management for chronic gastro-oesophageal reflux disease: UK collaborative randomised trial. BMJ 2008;337: [doi:10.1136/bmj.a2664].
24. Bowdler DA, Stell PM. Surgical management of posterior pharyngeal pulsion diverticulum: inversion versus one stage excision. Br J Surg 1987;74:988–90.
25. Payne WS, Clagett OT. Pharyngeal and esophageal diverticuli. Curr Probl Surg 1965;2:1–31.
26. Rizzetto C, Zaninotto G, Costantini M, et al. Zenker's diverticula: feasibility of a tailored approach based on diverticulum size. J Gastrointest Surg 2008; 12(12):2057–64.
27. Maffetton V, Renzi A, Brusciano L, et al. Laparoscopic approach in the treatment of epiphrenic diverticula: long-term results. Surg Endosc 2004; 18(5):741–5.
28. Katsinelos P, Chatzimavroudis G, Zavos C, et al. Long-term botulinum toxin treatment for dysphagia due to large epiphrenic diverticulum in elderly patients: a report of two cases. Dysphagia 2009; 24:109–13.
29. Miettinen M, Sarlomo-Rikala M, Lasota J. Gastrointestinal stromal tumors: recent advances in understanding of their biology [review]. Hum Pathol 1999;30(10):1213–20.
30. Jiang G, Zhao H, Yang F, et al. Thoracoscopic enucleation of esophageal leiomyoma: a retrospective study on 40 cases. Dis Esophagus 2009;22: 279–83.
31. Sandha GS, Marcon NE. Expandable metal stents for benign esophageal obstruction. Gastrointest Endosc Clin N Am 1999;9(3):437–46.
32. Ackroyd R, Watson DI, Devitt PG, et al. Expandable metallic stents should not be used in the treatment of benign esophageal strictures. J Gastroenterol Hepatol 2001;16(4):484–7.
33. Barthel JS, Kelley ST, Klapman JB. Management of persistent gastroesophageal anastomotic strictures with removable self-expandable polyester silicon-covered (Polyflex) stents: an alternative to serial dilation. Gastrointest Endosc 2008;67(3):546–52.
34. Triester SL, Fleischer DE, Sharma VK. Failure of self-expanding plastic stents in treatment of refractory benign esophageal strictures. Endoscopy 2006; 38(5):533–7.
35. Lyons WS, Seremetis MG, deGuzman VC, et al. Ruptures and perforations of the esophagus: the case for conservative supportive management. Ann Thorac Surg 1978;25:346.
36. Amir AI, van Dullemen H, Plukker JT. Selective approach in the treatment of esophageal perforations. Scand J Gastroenterol 2004;39:418–22.
37. Tuebergen D, Rijcken E, Mennigen R, et al. Treatment of thoracic esophageal anastomotic leaks and esophageal perforations with endoluminal stents: efficacy and current limitations. J Gastrointest Surg 2008; 12(7):1168–76.

Resection for Esophageal Cancer in the Elderly

Andrew C. Chang, MD[a,b,*], Julia S. Lee, MS[b]

KEYWORDS

• Esophagectomy • Mortality • Complications
• Older patient • Human

CANCER INCIDENCE AND MORTALITY

Esophageal cancer remains a highly lethal malignancy, with an annual death rate of 7.9/100,000 for men and 1.7/100,000 for women nearly matching its annual incidence of 7.9/100,000 for men and 1.8/100,000 for women. These rates have been increasing slowly across the entire United States population. Most cases of esophageal cancer occur in patients 65 years of age or older, with more than one third of incident cases and deaths affecting patients 75 years of age or older (**Fig. 1**).[1–3] Of the patients older than 65 years of age undergoing esophagectomy captured in the linked Surveillance, Epidemiology and End Results (SEER)-Medicare databases, 34% are 75 years old or older. Although esophageal resection remains the mainstay of treatment for patients who have potentially resectable carcinoma, patient age continues to be a major factor in clinical decision making.

The Worldwide Esophageal Cancer Collaborative recently evaluated survival among 4725 patients undergoing esophagectomy alone, without preoperative or adjuvant chemotherapy or radiation at 13 institutions worldwide.[4] In this study, the average patient age was 62 ± 11 years, and 75% of patients underwent esophagectomy in the 1990s and 2000s. Patient survival differed significantly and distinctively by all staging criteria including tumor, lymph node, metastasis stage, histology, grade, and number of involved lymph nodes. Demographically, the region of world and patient race were not determinants for patient survival. In this cohort of patients, increasing age was a significant adverse risk factor for overall long-term survival, with patients 70 years of age and older having worse survival than patients in younger deciles of age. Operative mortality varied from 0% to 7% among the institutions whose data were included in this study. Although this collaborative was assembled with the primary goal of developing a revised system for staging esophageal cancer, these international data, accumulated from specialized centers, suggest that patient age has a significant impact on early and long-term survival following esophagectomy for cancer, as discussed in this article.

Using the SEER-Medicare databases, Paulson and colleagues[5] identified the rate of resection in a study cohort of 2386 patients who had resectable (stage I, II, or III) esophageal cancer diagnosed between 1997 and 2002. In this cohort they found that 813 patients (34%) had received esophagectomy. Among other factors found to be associated with a lower likelihood for undergoing operation, including non-white race, residence in a high-poverty area, and a greater number of comorbidities, these authors found that increasing age was associated significantly with decreased likelihood of operation. Patients aged 75 to 79 years were half as likely to undergo esophagectomy as patients aged 65 to 74 years. Older patients who had stage II or stage III esophageal cancer, although generally considered resectable, also

[a] Section of General Thoracic Surgery, University of Michigan Health Systems, TC2120G/5344, 1500 East Medical Center Drive, Ann Arbor, MI 48109, USA
[b] Biostatistics Unit, Comprehensive Cancer Center, 300 North Ingalls Building, University of Michigan Health Systems, TC2120G/5344, 1500 East Medical Center Drive, Ann Arbor, MI 48109, USA
* Corresponding author. Section of General Thoracic Surgery, University of Michigan Health Systems, TC2120G/5344, 1500 East Medical Center Drive, Ann Arbor, MI 48109.
E-mail address: andrwchg@umich.edu (A.C. Chang).

Thorac Surg Clin 19 (2009) 333–343
doi:10.1016/j.thorsurg.2009.06.002
1547-4127/09/$ – see front matter

thoracic.theclinics.com

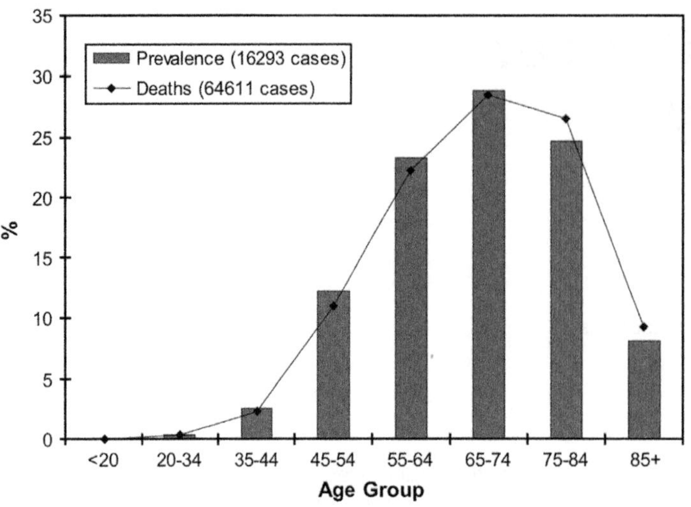

Fig. 1. Distribution of new cases of (*bar*) and deaths (*line*) caused by esophageal cancer among cohorts of age, 2001–2005, Surveillance, Epidemiology and End Results. (*Data from* Ries L, Melbert D, Krapcho M, et al. SEER cancer statistics review, 1975-2005, National Cancer Institute. Bethesda (MD), Available at: http://seer.cancer.gov/csr/1975_2005/, based on November 2007 SEER data submission, posted to the SEER web site 2008. Accessed February 1, 2009.)

were less likely than younger patients to undergo operation. Overall 5-year survival was significantly better for patients undergoing operation than for non-surgically treated patients (28% and 10% respectively), even after adjustment for patient and tumor characteristics, including age, comorbidity burden, socioeconomic region, race, and tumor stage (hazard ratio, 0.69; $P < .001$, Cox proportional hazards model). Although this study focused on the issue of health care disparities based on race and socioeconomic status, the findings also demonstrate that increasing patient age continues to be a determinant in the delivery of appropriate treatment, including esophagectomy, for patients who have esophageal cancer.

Similar findings can be gleaned from a population-based study of the National Cancer Registry, Ireland, in which the authors found that older patients were more likely to be referred for nonoperative management such as chemotherapy and/or radiation therapy, or to receive no treatment at all, rather than resection for curative intent. Among 3165 patients diagnosed with esophageal cancer from 1994 to 2001, 982 underwent resection, but, when compared with patients less than 60 years of age, the likelihood for resection was significantly lower among older cohorts by 33%, 74% and 93% for patients aged 60 to 69 years, 70 to 79 years, and 80 years and older, respectively. There was limited analysis of the reasons for this practice pattern, although the authors speculated that these differences might be attributed in part to the lack of centralized care and limited availability of specialized cancer services.[6]

MORTALITY: POPULATION-BASED DATA

Several population-based studies have demonstrated a consistent adverse effect of increasing age on mortality following esophagectomy. Using data obtained as part of the Department of Veterans Affairs (VA) National Surgical Quality Improvement Program (NSQIP),[7] Bailey and colleagues[8] identified 1777 patients undergoing esophagectomy, including 1509 (85%) for cancer between 1991 and 2000, at 109 VA Medical Centers. Overall mortality was 10%, and one or more perioperative complications occurred in nearly 50% of these patients. Although multivariate analysis found increasing age to be a significant risk factor in for both 30-day mortality and morbidity, limited data were published describing the age distribution of this study population. The odds ratio for mortality was 1.05, indicating a 5% increased risk of 30-day mortality for every increasing year of age. A diagnosis of malignancy did not present an increased risk for 30-day mortality or for complications in the study population.

Using the Swedish national cancer registry, Rouvelas and colleagues[9] identified 764 patients undergoing resection alone for esophageal carcinoma from 1987 to 2000, including 302 patients aged 66 to 75 years and 140 patients aged 75 years or older. Overall 30-day mortality was 7.3%. Although older patients were at greater risk for mortality, this trend was not statistically significant with a hazard ratio of 1.28 (95% confidence interval 0.96–1.72) for patients 75 years or greater.

Cronin-Fenton and colleagues[6] from the National Cancer Registry, Ireland, identified 3165 patients diagnosed as having esophageal cancer or gastroesophageal junction carcinomas from 1994 to 2001, including 1026 patients (32%) aged 70 to 79 years and 665 patients (21%) aged 80 years or older. In this sample, 982 patients (31%) underwent cancer-directed operation including 611 patients for esophageal carcinoma and 316 patients for gastroesophageal carcinoma. Data regarding associated comorbidities at the time of diagnosis were not available in this registry. Although 30-day mortality was increased by nearly 50% among patients older than 70 years compared with younger patients, this trend was not statistically significant (hazard ratio, 1.49, 95% confidence interval, 0.95–2.33). Overall, long-term survival was significantly worse among older patients (hazard ratio, 1.52, 95% confidence interval, 1.28–1.80).

Population-based administrative databases in the United States have provided a broad perspective of outcomes following esophagectomy, allowing evaluation of effects caused by a variety of factors, including hospital teaching status, geographic region, and socioeconomic status. Early studies demonstrated a significant relationship between case volume and outcomes at both the hospital[10,11] and surgeon[12] level that has led to a general inquiry into the structures and processes of care that might be important determinants of the volume–outcome relationship.[13,14] Analyses of these databases also provide more insight into the outcomes of infrequently performed operations, such as esophagectomy, in older patients.

Finlayson and colleagues[15] accessed the Health Care Financing Administration's Medicare Provider Analysis and Review and Denominator files for 1994 to 1999 and found that early mortality among 4080 patients aged 65 to 99 years undergoing esophagectomy was 13.6%. When this study population was stratified by age cohorts, mortality ranged from 10.7% for the youngest cohort of patients aged 65 to 69 years to 18.9% or greater for patients 80 years or older. Using a broader study population of 5282 patients obtained from the all-payer 1995 to 1997 Nationwide Inpatient Sample, representative of an estimated 20% of the United States population, Finlayson and colleagues[16] observed that operative mortality was 8.1% among patients 65 years of age or older undergoing operation at high-volume hospitals (where more than nine esophagectomies were performed annually), compared with 19.3% at low-volume hospitals (where fewer than four esophagectomies were performed annually) (adjusted odds ratio, 0.38, 95% confidence interval 0.24–0.62). Among patients younger than 65 years of age, hospital volume did not seem to be a significant factor for operative mortality.

These investigators explored the early and long-term outcomes of esophagectomy in a larger sample of 27,957 patients, 65 years old or older, from the 1994 to 2003 Nationwide Inpatient Sample, including 15,145 patients (54.2%) aged 70 to 79 years and 3150 patients (11.3%) age 80 years and older.[17] In this sample the frequency of patients with two or more comorbid conditions increased significantly in the older age cohorts, from 58.0% in patients 65 to 69 years of age to 61.7% in patients 70 to 79 years of age and 65.0% in patients age 80 years and older. Operative mortality (defined as death before hospital discharge) was significantly different and increased with each age cohort, from 8.8% to 13.4% and to 19.9%, respectively ($P < .0001$).

Patient functional status in this cohort was determined by patient discharge status. Compared with 83.5% of patients 65 to 69 years of age, significantly fewer patients in the older cohorts (74.6% and 54.2%, respectively) ($P <$ .0001) were discharged to home. Instead, 42% of patients 80 years or older were discharged to a skilled nursing facility or other type of long-term care facility, compared with 14.2% of patients 65 to 69 years of age.

Long-term survival was determined in a second analytic cohort using the 1992 to 2001 SEER-Medicare–linked databases, representing approximately 14% of the United States population. Overall 5-year survival was significantly worse among octogenarians undergoing esophagectomy than in patients between 65 and 69 years of age (**Fig. 2**), although these data were derived from only 216 patients identified in the SEER-Medicare–linked databases.

Although such studies can carry greater statistical power and capture outcomes across the spectrum of hospital and provider systems on a scale that might not be feasible in most single-center reports, administrative databases, even when linked to cancer registries, lack the clinical detail that permits better understanding of the underlying processes and structures of care that are likely determinants of patient outcomes, particularly for esophagectomy.[18] Population-wide studies based on administrative databases should be interpreted with caution and should be used for purposes of hypothesis development, rather than for policy implementation, particularly if applied to specific patient cohorts such as the elderly.

MORTALITY: CENTER-SPECIFIC REPORTS

Poon and colleagues[19] have demonstrated that increasing age remains a significant risk factor for operative (30-day) mortality but should not be the only factor considered in decision making concerning resection. In a retrospective evaluation of 737 patients, including 167 patients 70 years or older, undergoing esophagectomy for carcinoma from 1982 to 1996, they observed significantly

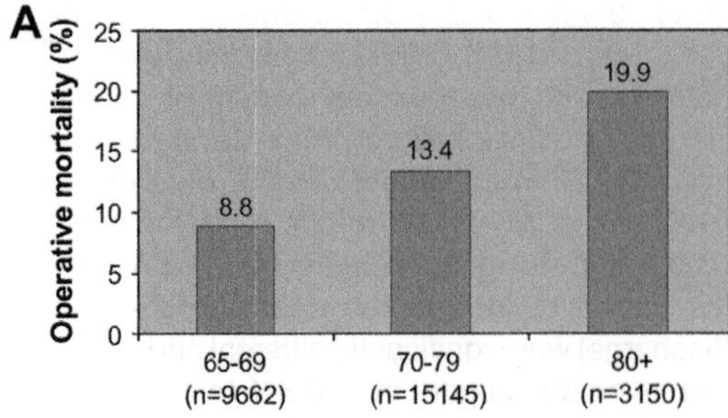

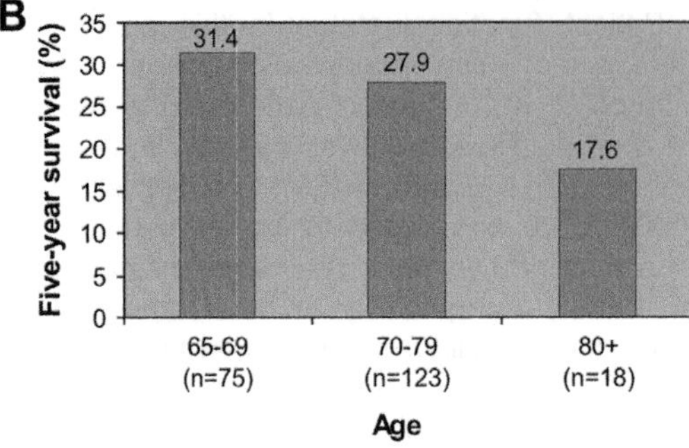

Fig. 2. (*A*) Operative mortality following esophagectomy (1994–2003 nationwide inpatient sample). (*B*) Overall 5-year survival following esophagectomy for cancer (1992–2001 SEER-Medicare–linked data base). (*Data from* Finlayson E, Fan Z, Birkmeyer JD. Outcomes in octogenarians undergoing high-risk cancer operation: a national study. J Am Coll Surg 2007;205:729–34; with permission.)

increased ($P < .02$) operative mortality of 7.2% among patients 70 years or older, compared with 3.0% in younger patients. In the older group, 25% (42 patients) received a transhiatal approach compared with 12% (71 patients) of younger patients. Despite this higher operative mortality, hospital mortality (designated as occurring during the same hospitalization up to 6 months following operation) did not differ significantly, occurring in 18.0% of the older patients and in 14.4% of the younger group of patients. Overall long-term survival was significantly worse ($P < .01$) among older patients, who had median 5-year survival times and survival rates of 16 months and 26%, respectively, compared with 33 months and 35%, respectively, in the younger cohort. When non–cancer-related deaths were censored from analysis, long-term survival was equivalent, with median 5-year survival times and rates of 28 months and 32%, respectively, in patients 70 years or older and 37 months and 37%, respectively, in younger patients.

In a separate report evaluating 434 patients undergoing esophagectomy for esophageal squamous cell carcinoma from 1990 to 2002, this group has observed that patient age did not seem to differ among patients with or without technical complications, defined as anastomotic leak, recurrent laryngeal nerve palsy, chylothorax, conduit ischemic necrosis, postoperative hemorrhage requiring reoperation, wound dehiscence, or delayed gastric emptying.[20]

In a series of 773 patients who had esophageal cancer and underwent esophagectomy from 1990 to 2003, more than 95% of whom received thoracotomy, Abunasra and colleagues[21] found that operative (30-day) and hospital mortality occurred in 4.8% (37 patients). When this study population was divided into quartiles by age, those in the oldest cohort, aged 73 years and older, were at more than four times greater risk for operative mortality than patients aged 60 years or less. When analyzed as a continuous variable, each year of increasing age carried an odds ratio of 1.07 (95% confidence interval, 1.02–1.12), indicating a nearly doubled risk of early mortality for each decade of increasing age. Other risk factors included obstructive lung disease and cervical or upper-third esophageal tumor location.

Moskovitz and colleagues[22] reported a single-center experience evaluating 751 patients, 50 years or older, undergoing esophagectomy between 1996 and 2005. Younger patients, who had fewer comorbidities and lower perioperative mortality than patients aged 50 years or older, were excluded from this analysis to avoid any bias resulting from improved outcomes in this generally lower-risk population. Four percent of these patients (31 patients) were octogenarians, and 10% (76 patients) were age 75 to 79 years. Overall, 75% of patients underwent thoracotomy; slightly fewer thoracotomies were performed in octogenarians, but this difference was not statistically significant. Postoperative mortality, defined as 60-day or in-hospital mortality, was significantly increased in these older cohorts, with mortality of 19.4% in the octogenarian cohort, compared with 5.1% for the entire study cohort (hazard ratio, 3.9; $P < .01$; 95% confidence interval, 1.5–10.6). Although intraoperative blood loss and rates of perioperative complication (pulmonary, cardiovascular, infection, anastomotic leak) did not differ significantly between the younger and older cohorts in the study, older patients had longer hospital lengths of stay. Longer-term overall survival also was significantly worse among octogenarians, who had a median survival of 17 months compared with 47 months among 637 patients aged 50 to 75 years. These authors concluded that advanced age remains a significant risk factor for perioperative mortality and diminished long-term survival, independent of patient comorbidities. Although older patients had similar rates of perioperative complication, their hospital mortality and lengths of stay were increased, leading the authors to suggest that older patients have less physiologic reserve and capacity to survive these complications, consistent with findings from an earlier report from this group. In contrast to the findings of Ferri and colleagues,[20] Rizk and colleagues[23] found that patients older than 75 years experienced worse 30-day and 1-year survival if their operation was associated with perioperative complication, with a hazard ratio of 0.61 (95% confidence interval, 0.43–0.81) for patients without perioperative complication. These and earlier findings are listed **Table 1**.

In a previous report of outcomes in patients undergoing esophagectomy at the University of Michigan Health Systems between 1976 and 2006, the present authors found that both hospital mortality and operative blood loss decreased significantly between early and later eras of this overall experience.[24] During the last 15 years at this institution (1993–2008), reflecting more recent experience, 1251 patients, including 620 patients aged 65 years or older, have undergone esophagectomy for esophageal cancer. Transhiatal esophagectomy without thoracotomy was performed in 1212 patients (97%). Overall 30-day and hospital mortality was 2.6%, with no differences noted between younger and older patient cohorts. When evaluated by decade of age, overall long-term survival was significantly worse for patients 65 years of age or older than for the younger age cohorts (**Fig. 3**). Cox proportional hazards analysis in this population indicated that increasing age at operation was a significant risk factor for worse overall survival with hazard ratio of 1.022 (95% confidence interval, 1.014–1.031). Increasing age at operation remained a significant adverse risk factor for disease-specific survival, although to a lesser degree, with hazard ratio of 1.012 (95% confidence interval, 1.001–1.022) per year of increasing age, respectively (unpublished data).

Although considerable debate continues regarding the relative risks and benefits of esophageal resection with or without thoracotomy, whether operation approach influences perioperative outcomes or long-term survival in older patients is not well studied. Single-center reports such as those discussed earlier in this article and elsewhere[25–31] reinforce the opinion that operation approach does not seem to influence outcomes, including long-term survival, following esophagectomy in older patients.

OVERALL COMPLICATIONS

Few studies have sought expressly to evaluate patient age as a risk factor for postoperative complication following esophagectomy. Evaluation of the Swedish esophageal cancer registry identified 275 patients undergoing esophagectomy between 2001 and 2003, including 112 patients 70 years of age or older. In the entire study cohort, 46% experienced one or more complications, including anastomotic leak (9%), pulmonary complications (18%), cardiac, hepatic, or renal complications (17%), or technical complications such as intraoperative bleeding, recurrent laryngeal nerve injury, or need for reoperation (9%). Patients treated with preoperative chemotherapy and/or radiation therapy had a slightly increased complication rate that was not statistically significant. Although patient age was not a significant risk factor for the development of postoperative complications, patients who sustained multiple (three or more) postoperative complications were more likely to be older.[32]

Several single-center studies have reported differing conclusions regarding the association between age, perioperative complication, and mortality following esophagectomy for cancer. Atkins and colleagues[33] identified 379 patients undergoing esophagectomy including 341 patients who underwent resection for cancer between 1996 and 2002. Operative (30-day) mortality was 5.8%, with at least one complication occurring in 64% of patients. Multivariate analysis indicated that only increasing age and occurrence of pneumonia were risk factors for increased operative mortality, although in univariate analysis dysphagia, anastomotic leak, and increased comorbidities also were found to be associated significantly with operative mortality.

In contrast to a subsequent report from the same institution[21] (discussed earlier in this article), Alexiou and colleagues[34] found that increasing age alone did not have a significant adverse impact on perioperative complications, operative mortality, or long-term survival among 523 patients undergoing esophagectomy. Notably, a significantly greater proportion of older patients was found to be unfit for operation. In this study, 686 patients had been assessed for operation between 1987 and 1997; nearly 20% of the older patients (age 80–86 years) who were evaluated were excluded from operation, whereas only 2% of the patients aged less than 70 years and 5% of those aged 70–79 years were found to be inoperable. When patients undergoing operation were stratified by these deciles of age, no significant differences were observed in terms of

Table 1
Impact of patient age on outcomes following esophageal resection for cancer, selected recent studies

Author	Study Period, Data Source	Age Cohorts	Study Population	Operative Mortality (%)	Five-year Survival	Overall Survival, Adjusted Hazard Ratio[a]	*P*
Bailey et al (2003)[8]	1991–2000 VA-NSQIP	Continuum	1777 (1509 cancer)	9.8		1.05/year	0
Rouvelas et al (2005)[9]	1987–2000	<55	104		27.4	1.00 (reference)	
	Cancer Registry,	55–65	218		26.0	1.08 (0.82–1.42)	NS
	Sweden	66–75	302		25.0	1.01 (0.84–1.41)	NS
		>75	140		22.8		NS
Cronin-Fenton et al (2007)[6]	1994–2001	<70	No surgery: 1705			1.00 (reference)	0.99
	Cancer Registry,	70+				1.00 (0.89–1.12)	
	Ireland	<70	Resection: 927			1.00 (reference)	<0.001
		70+				1.52 (1.28–1.80)	
Finlayson et al (2007)[17]	1994–2003	65–69	9662	6.7			
	NIS	70–79	15145	9.3			
		80+	3150	15.5			<0.0001
	1992–2001	65–69	75		31.4		
	SEER-Medicare	70–79	123		27.9		
		80+	18		17.6		0.02
Poon et al (1998)[19]	1982–1996	<70	570	3.0	35.0		<0.02/<0.01
	Clinical database	70+	167	7.2	26.0		
Alexiou et al (1998)[24]	1987–1997	<70	337	4.7	25.1		NS
	Clinical database	70–79	150	6.7	21.2		
		80–86	36	5.6	19.8		

Study	Period / Source	Age group	n	Mortality (%)	Survival	Hazard ratio[a]	P
Abunasra et al (2005)[21]	1990–2003	<59.5	193	2.1		1.0 (reference)	0.01
	Clinical database	59.5–67.8	193	3.6		2.06 (0.52–8.22)	
		67.9–73.2	194	4.1		1.55 (0.36–6.72)	
		> 73.2	193	9.3		4.87 (1.35–17.55)	
Moskovitz et al (2006)[22]	1996–2005	<50	107	1.9		1.0 (reference)	
	Clinical database	50–59	228	4.8			
		60–70	285	5.6			
		70–79	207	7.3			
		80+	31	19.4		3.9 (1.5–10.6)	<0.01
					Median survival (months):		
		50–75			46.7		
		75–79			29.1		
		80+			16.8		0.01
					Five-year survival (%):		
Current report (2009)	1993–2008	Continuum	1251	2.6	39.7	1.022/year	<0.0001
	Clinical database	<55	241	0.8	59 (95% CI: 41, 55)		
		55–64	390	3.3	42 (36, 48)		
		65–74	418	2.2	38 (33, 43)		
		≥75	202	4.0	28 (21, 35)		

Abbreviations: NIS, Nationwide inpatient sample; NS, Not significant.

[a] Adjusted hazard ratios include 95% confidence interval.

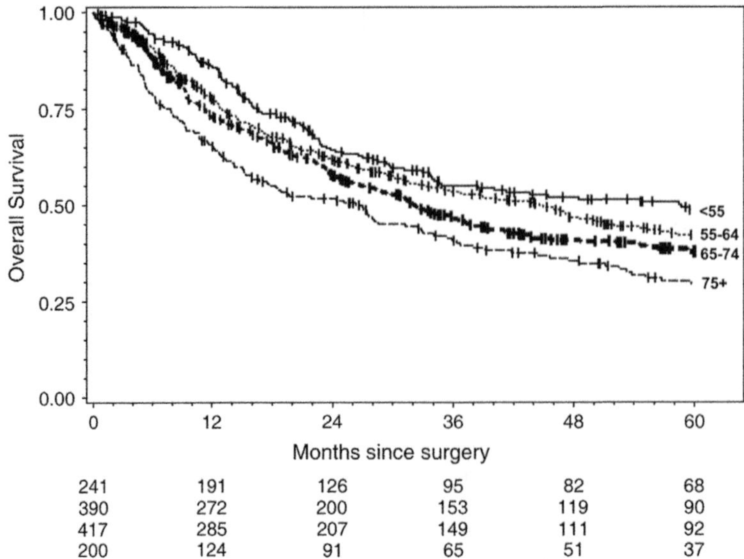

Fig. 3. Kaplan-Meier overall survival following esophagectomy for esophageal cancer, stratified by patient age, at the University of Michigan, 1993–2008.

perioperative complication or early mortality. Moreover, because long-term survival was equivalent among the different age cohorts, the authors concluded that among highly selected older patients the survival benefit of esophageal resection can be similar to that in younger counterparts, as had been suggested by others.[19]

POSTOPERATIVE DELIRIUM

Postoperative delirium occurs in approximately 10% to 15% of patients undergoing non-cardiac general surgery,[35,36] including esophagectomy,[37] and ranges as high as 50% or greater, particularly in older patients.[38] Delirium has been associated with other major postoperative complications, particularly myocardial infarction, pneumonia, pulmonary edema, and respiratory failure. Moreover, delirium seems to increase both hospital and intermediate-term mortality as well as the likelihood of transfer to long-term care.[39] Although there are limited data evaluating the impact of delirium in older patients following esophagectomy, risk factors for the development of postoperative delirium following non-cardiac surgery include an age of 70 years or older, poor cognitive or functional status, self-reported alcohol abuse, and abnormal preoperative serum sodium, potassium, or glucose levels.[35] Additionally, factors during hospitalization such as use of physical restraints, malnutrition, use of a bladder catheter, the addition of three or more medications, and adverse outcomes from iatrogenic events can precipitate postoperative delirium, particularly among patients who have predisposing risks for delirium.[36,40] These factors have been used to create risk profiles for hospitalized general medicine patients and for patients undergoing abdominal or thoracic operation[39,41] but remain to be validated among patients undergoing esophageal resection.

QUALITY OF LIFE

In evaluating an operation designed to preserve the ability to eat and also to provide satisfactory and durable oncologic outcomes, formal assessment of postoperative quality of life has been largely qualitative, and there are few reports evaluating quality of life following esophagectomy for carcinoma in older patients. Using the Medical Outcomes Study 36-Item Short-Form Health Survey (MOS SF-36), Deschamps[42] evaluated postoperative measures of quality of life in eight areas: general health (health perception), daily activities (physical functioning), work (role - physical), emotional problems (role - emotional), social activities (social functioning), nervousness/depression (mental health), pain (bodily pain), and vitality (energy/fatigue). After esophagectomy for Barrett's esophagus with high-grade dysplasia, older patients were more likely to report diminished physical function and performance at work, compared with the national standard. In contrast, among patients undergoing resection for carcinoma, although self-perception of physical functioning was significantly diminished in this entire cohort, patient age was not associated with any significant decline in the eight areas assessed by the MOS SF-36.

It behooves the operating surgeon to assure that patients receive thorough preoperative education regarding the potential risks and benefits of esophageal resection and to obtain informed patient consent. Following operation and after medical recovery, subsequent discussions regarding prognostic implications of the operative findings might be tempered by patient preference, although this approach has not been established for patients undergoing esophagectomy. In a recent survey-based analysis of patient preferences for disclosure of prognostic information, patient age did not influence the predominant desire for a detailed discussion of potential outcomes and treatment options. The majority of patients (80%) preferred that their surgeon start the discussion regarding prognosis, but patients who wished to initiate the discussion themselves or to defer the discussion completely were significantly older (median age, 69 years versus 60 years).[43]

SUMMARY

Although studies differ in their definition of the older patient, increasing age, when considered as a continuum, is associated with greater operative mortality. Complication rates also seem to be significantly higher with advancing age, possibly because of limited physiologic reserve. As the understanding of risk factors for perioperative morbidity and mortality following esophagectomy has improved, investigators have sought to develop models for risk stratification[44–46] in which patient age is a significant but not the sole determinant of prospective assessment of risk for complication or mortality. Such prognostic indicators, if validated among independent patient cohorts, can serve as useful adjuncts in decision making with appropriate clinical judgment.

In addition, reported patient survival differs dramatically between rates reported by single centers and rates observed in population-based studies, with operative mortality rates typically lower in single-center reports. Although such reports usually are issued from groups with higher operative volume that might be a surrogate for surgical experience, it also is possible that the association between operation volume and improved outcomes reflects optimization of institution-specific infrastructure and/or clinical care pathways.[37] As these processes of care evolve, they should be tailored with attention to differences in the care of older patients who have esophageal cancer. Whether widespread application of such processes of care then can lead to less perioperative mortality and fewer complications and to improved long-term survival remains untested.

ACKNOWLEDGMENTS

The authors thank Dr. Mark B Orringer for his critical comments.

REFERENCES

1. Birkmeyer JD, Sun Y, Wong SL, et al. Hospital volume and late survival after cancer surgery. Ann Surg 2007;245(5):777–83.
2. Ries L, Melbert D, Krapcho M, et al. SEER cancer statistics review, 1975-2005. Available at: http://seer.cancer.gov/csr/1975_2005/. based on November 2007 SEER data submission, posted to the SEER web site, 2008. Accessed February 1, 2009.
3. Chang AC, Ji H, Birkmeyer NJ, et al. Outcomes after transhiatal and transthoracic esophagectomy for cancer. Ann Thorac Surg 2008;85(2):424–9.
4. Rice TW, Rusch VW, Apperson-Hansen C, et al. Worldwide esophageal cancer collaboration. Dis Esophagus 2009;22(1):1–8.
5. Paulson EC, Ra J, Armstrong K, et al. Underuse of esophagectomy as treatment for resectable esophageal cancer. Arch Surg 2008;143(12):1198–203.
6. Cronin-Fenton DP, Sharp L, Carsin AE, et al. Patterns of care and effects on mortality for cancers of the oesophagus and gastric cardia: a population-based study. Eur J Cancer 2007;43(3):565–75.
7. Khuri SF, Daley J, Henderson W, et al. The Department of Veterans Affairs' NSQIP: the first national, validated, outcome-based, risk-adjusted, and peer-controlled program for the measurement and enhancement of the quality of surgical care. Ann Surg 1998;228(4):491–507.
8. Bailey SH, Bull DA, Harpole DH, et al. Outcomes after esophagectomy: a ten-year prospective cohort. Ann Thorac Surg 2003;75(1):217–22.
9. Rouvelas I, Zeng W, Lindblad M, et al. Survival after surgery for oesophageal cancer: a population-based study. Lancet Oncol 2005;6(11):864–70.
10. Begg CB, Cramer LD, Hoskins WJ, et al. Impact of hospital volume on operative mortality for major cancer surgery. JAMA 1998;280(20):1747–51.
11. Birkmeyer JD, Siewers AE, Finlayson EVA, et al. Hospital volume and surgical mortality in the United States. N Engl J Med 2002;346(15):1128–37.
12. Birkmeyer JD, Stukel TA, Siewers AE, et al. Surgeon volume and operative mortality in the United States. N Engl J Med 2003;349(22):2117–27.
13. Birkmeyer JD, Sun Y, Goldfaden A, et al. Volume and process of care in high-risk cancer surgery. Cancer 2006;106(11):2476–81.
14. Meguid RA, Weiss ES, Chang DC, et al. The effect of volume on esophageal cancer resections: what

constitutes acceptable resection volumes for centers of excellence? J Thorac Cardiovasc Surg 2009;137(1):23–9.

15. Finlayson EV, Birkmeyer JD. Operative mortality with elective surgery in older adults. Eff Clin Pract 2001; 4(4):172–7.
16. Finlayson EV, Goodney PP, Birkmeyer JD. Hospital volume and operative mortality in cancer surgery: a national study. Arch Surg 2003;138(7):721–5.
17. Finlayson E, Fan Z, Birkmeyer JD. Outcomes in octogenarians undergoing high-risk cancer operation: a national study. J Am Coll Surg 2007;205(6): 729–34.
18. Kozower BD, Stukenborg GJ, Lau CL, et al. Measuring the quality of surgical outcomes in general thoracic surgery: should surgical volume be used to direct patient referrals? Ann Thorac Surg 2008;86(5):1405–8.
19. Poon RT, Law SY, Chu KM, et al. Esophagectomy for carcinoma of the esophagus in the elderly: results of current surgical management. Ann Surg 1998; 227(3):357–64.
20. Ferri LE, Law S, Wong KH, et al. The influence of technical complications on postoperative outcome and survival after esophagectomy. Ann Surg Oncol 2006;13(4):557–64.
21. Abunasra H, Lewis S, Beggs L, et al. Predictors of operative death after oesophagectomy for carcinoma. Br J Surg 2005;92(8):1029–33.
22. Moskovitz AH, Rizk NP, Venkatraman E, et al. Mortality increases for octogenarians undergoing esophagogastrectomy for esophageal cancer. Ann Thorac Surg 2006;82(6):2031–6.
23. Rizk NP, Bach PB, Schrag D, et al. The impact of complications on outcomes after resection for esophageal and gastroesophageal junction carcinoma. J Am Coll Surg 2004;198(1):42–50.
24. Orringer MB, Marshall B, Chang AC, et al. Two thousand transhiatal esophagectomies: changing trends, lessons learned. Ann Surg 2007;246(3): 363–72.
25. Nigro JJ, DeMeester SR, Hagen JA, et al. Node status in transmural esophageal adenocarcinoma and outcome after en bloc esophagectomy. J Thorac Cardiovasc Surg 1999;117(5):960–8.
26. Hulscher JBF, van Sandick JW, Tijssen JGP, et al. The recurrence pattern of esophageal carcinoma after transhiatal resection. J Am Coll Surg 2000; 191(2):143–8.
27. Hulscher JBF, van Sandick JW, de Boer AGEM, et al. Extended transthoracic resection compared with limited transhiatal resection for adenocarcinoma of the esophagus. N Engl J Med 2002; 347(21):1662–9.
28. McCulloch P, Ward J, Tekkis PP. Mortality and morbidity in gastro-oesophageal cancer surgery: initial results of ASCOT multicentre prospective cohort study. Br Med J 2003; 327(7425):1192–7.
29. Rentz J, Bull D, Harpole D, et al. Transthoracic versus transhiatal esophagectomy: a prospective study of 945 patients. J Thorac Cardiovasc Surg 2003;125(5):1114–20.
30. Gockel I, Heckhoff S, Messow C, et al. Transhiatal and transthoracic resection in adenocarcinoma of the esophagus: does the operative approach have an influence on the long-term prognosis? World J Surg Oncol 2005;3(1):40.
31. Yekebas EF, Schurr PG, Kaifi JT, et al. Effectiveness of radical en-bloc-esophagectomy compared to transhiatal esophagectomy in squamous cell cancer of the esophagus is influenced by nodal micrometastases. J Surg Oncol 2006;93(7):541–9.
32. Viklund P, Lindblad M, Lu M, et al. Risk factors for complications after esophageal cancer resection: a prospective population-based study in Sweden. Ann Surg 2006;243(2):204–11.
33. Atkins BZ, Shah AS, Hutcheson KA, et al. Reducing hospital morbidity and mortality following esophagectomy. Ann Thorac Surg 2004;78(4): 1170–6.
34. Alexiou C, Beggs D, Salama FD, et al. Surgery for esophageal cancer in elderly patients: the view from Nottingham. J Thorac Cardiovasc Surg 1998; 116(4):545–53.
35. Marcantonio ER, Goldman L, Mangione CM, et al. A clinical prediction rule for delirium after elective noncardiac surgery. JAMA 1994;271(2):134–9.
36. Anderson D. Preventing delirium in older people. Br Med Bull 2005;73–74(1):25–34.
37. Low D, Kunz S, Schembre D, et al. Esophagectomy—it's not just about mortality anymore: standardized perioperative clinical pathways improve outcomes in patients with esophageal cancer. J Gastrointest Surg 2007;11(11):1395–402.
38. Flinn DR, Diehl KM, Seyfried LS, et al. Prevention, diagnosis and management of post-operative delirium in older adults. J Am Coll Surg 2009; 209(2):261–8 [quiz: 294].
39. Robinson TN, Raeburn CD, Tran ZV, et al. Postoperative delirium in the elderly: risk factors and outcomes. Ann Surg 2009;249(1):173–8.
40. Inouye SK, Charpentier PA. Precipitating factors for delirium in hospitalized elderly persons. Predictive model and interrelationship with baseline vulnerability. JAMA 1996;275(11):852–7.
41. Ganai S, Lee KF, Merrill A, et al. Adverse outcomes of geriatric patients undergoing abdominal surgery who are at high risk for delirium. Arch Surg 2007; 142(11):1072–8.
42. Deschamps C, Nichols FC 3rd, Cassivi SD, et al. Long-term function and quality of life after esophageal resection for cancer and Barrett's. Surg Clin North Am 2005;85(3):649–56. xi.

43. Lagarde S, Franssen S, van Werven J, et al. Patient preferences for the disclosure of prognosis after esophagectomy for cancer with curative intent. Ann Surg Oncol 2008;15(11): 3289–98.
44. Aust JB, Henderson W, Khuri S, et al. The impact of operative complexity on patient risk factors. Ann Surg 2005;241(6):1024–7.
45. Shende MR, Waxman J, Luketich JD. Predictive ability of preoperative indices for esophagectomy. Thorac Surg Clin 2007;17(3):337–41.
46. Lagarde SM, Reitsma JB, Maris A-KD, et al. Preoperative prediction of the occurrence and severity of complications after esophagectomy for cancer with use of a nomogram. Ann Thorac Surg 2008;85(6): 1938–45.

The Emerging Role of Minimally Invasive Surgical Techniques for the Treatment of Lung Malignancy in the Elderly

Paul M. Heerdt, MD, PhD[a,b,*], Bernard J. Park, MD[c]

KEYWORDS

• Aging • Lung cancer • VATS

Although cancer can occur at any age, it disproportionately strikes the elderly, with persons older than 65 years exhibiting a 9.8-fold higher incidence compared with a younger population.[1] Demographic projections now indicate that by the year 2030, the number of United States citizens older than 65 years will double to a projected 70 million, with those older than 80 years making up 5.4% of the total population.[2] Consistent with the age-related incidence of cancer and the overall aging of the population is an increase in the absolute number of elderly patients presenting with potentially resectable malignancy.

For lung cancer in particular, approximately 175,000 patients per year in the United States are diagnosed with bronchogenic carcinoma, with a median age at diagnosis now in excess of 70 years.[3] For non–small cell lung cancer (NSCLC), which accounts for roughly 80% of pulmonary malignancy, anatomic resection (lobectomy) remains the best curative option for early-stage disease. There is, however, a clear association between advanced age and perioperative morbidity and mortality.[4] Accordingly, there is increasing interest in applying minimally invasive surgical techniques in elderly patients requiring lobectomy because of the belief that it will improve outcome. The purpose of this review is to examine the available data regarding this belief.

THE RISK/BENEFIT RELATIONSHIP OF SURGICAL INTERVENTION FOR LUNG CANCER IN THE ELDERLY

Compared with a younger patient, an elderly person may have different therapeutic goals when the inherent surgical risks of thoracotomy and lung resection are considered in the context of comorbid conditions and the potential disparity between chronologic and physiologic age (ie, the wide range of physical and mental capacity). For patients 80 years and older, data from the Lung Cancer Study Group published in 1983 indicated that complication rates and mortality were substantially higher than for patients younger than 65 years (30-day mortality rate of 8.1% versus 1.6%).[5] Recent studies, however, have suggested improved survival following lung

A version of this article originally appeared in the June 2008 issue of Anesthesiology Clinics.

[a] Departments of Anesthesiology and Pharmacology, Weill Medical College of Cornell University, 1300 York Avenue, LC-206, New York, NY 10021, USA

[b] Department of Anesthesiology and Critical Care Medicine, Memorial Sloan-Kettering Cancer Center, 1275 York Avenue, New York, NY 10021, USA

[c] Department of Surgery, Division of Thoracic Surgery, Memorial Sloan-Kettering Cancer Center, 1275 York Avenue, New York, NY 10021, USA

* Corresponding author. 1300 York Avenue, LC-206, New York, NY 10021.

E-mail address: pmheerd@med.cornell.edu (P.M. Heerdt).

Thorac Surg Clin 19 (2009) 345–351

doi:10.1016/j.thorsurg.2009.06.006

1547-4127/09/$ – see front matter

resection in octogenarians. For example, a 1998 report of 7099 operations over 1 year in Japan noted 30-day mortality rates after thoracotomy and lung resection of 0.4% for patients younger than 60 years, 1.3% for those aged 60 to 69 years, 2.0% for those aged 70 to 79 years, and 2.2% for those 80 years and older (225 of the 7099 cases).[6] For patients older than 70 years, Birim and colleagues[7] found a hospital mortality rate of 3.2% in a retrospective study of 126 consecutive patients and concluded that operative mortality is low enough to justify pulmonary resection for lung cancer in this population.

Despite data suggesting somewhat favorable survival statistics, many elderly patients remain concerned about the potential for consequences and complications that would prolong hospitalization and possibly persist following discharge, thus limiting their independence. Accordingly, long-term survival may become less important than relief of symptoms and maintaining their preoperative level of function. These concerns are not without merit. For example, in a recent retrospective review covering a 22-year experience in patients 80 years and older who had stage I NSCLC, Brock and colleagues[8] reported that 44% experienced one or more postoperative complications, most of which were cardiopulmonary. Other investigators reported morbidity rates ranging from 20% to 60%[9–13] in patients older than 80 years. Ultimately, elderly patients may not be inclined to accept the risks of major surgery, even if it might be curative, in favor of less invasive alternatives;[14] however, data indicate that for patients older than 75 years who have stage I or II NSCLC and opt for nonsurgical treatment, most deaths will be related to the progression of lung cancer rather than to other causes.[15] It is within this context that less extensive and less invasive procedures become attractive options to elderly patients.

THE EMERGING ROLE OF MINIMALLY INVASIVE SURGICAL TECHNIQUES

Although it is clearly beneficial for institutions and clinicians to offer less invasive approaches for the surgical treatment of lung cancer—and patients are appropriately drawn to the prospect of less postoperative pain and faster recovery—it is important to first consider what "less invasive" or "minimally invasive" means and whether the techniques are oncologically equivalent to standard thoracotomy. Given the association between the magnitude of pulmonary resection and postoperative complications in elderly patients, some surgeons advocate less extensive lung-sparing techniques such as wedge resection and segmentectomy whenever possible.[16] Although controversy exists as to whether these procedures, which still involve at least a limited thoracotomy, carry a higher risk of local recurrence, Mery and colleagues,[17] using data from the Surveillance, Epidemiology, and End Results database, found that, among patients 75 years and older, there was no difference in overall survival between patients undergoing lobectomy and those undergoing limited resection.

The scientific literature and the lay press contain a wide variety of publications relating video-assisted thoracoscopic surgery (VATS) as a truly minimally invasive approach to the treatment of lung cancer. Published data suggest that relative to thoracotomy, VATS patients experience shorter postoperative hospital stays, lower narcotic requirements for postoperative pain, and reduced shoulder dysfunction.[18] Similarly, patients who undergo VATS lobectomy report less postoperative pain, decreased time until return to preoperative activities, and higher satisfaction with the results of surgery than patients undergoing conventional thoracotomy.[19] In addition, there is a lower observed incidence of postoperative confusion,[20] which has been associated with increased postoperative morbidity and mortality. A recent review of 1100 VATS lobectomies with lymph node sampling or dissection in patients who had a mean age of 71.2 years demonstrated low rates of mortality (< 1%) and morbidity, with 84.7% of patients exhibiting no significant complications.[21]

When considering the published scientific data and the promotional literature disseminated to the public, it is important to understand exactly what is meant by "VATS lobectomy." Careful examination of the described methods reveals variation in the technique among experienced practitioners, particularly with regard to the number of access ports used for insertion of a camera and instruments, and the size and manipulation (ie, use of a mechanical rib-spreader) of the utility incision used for instrument insertion and removal of the specimen.[22] Recently, in an effort to standardize the approach to VATS lobectomy, the Cancer and Leukemia Group B reported results of a prospective trial to elucidate its feasibility for early NSCLC.[23] The standard definition for VATS lobectomy included (1) videoscopic guidance, (2) the use of one 4- to 8-cm access and two 0.5-cm port incisions without rib spreading, and (3) pulmonary lobectomy by way of traditional individual hilar dissection and ligation. Using this "standard" definition, the investigators were able to demonstrate acceptable perioperative results.

Questions remain as to whether lobectomy by way of thoracotomy and VATS is an equivalent therapeutic intervention for cancer despite favorable perioperative outcome data. A series of 159 VATS lobectomies for stage I and stage II NSCLC revealed long-term outcomes and local recurrence rates that were at least equivalent to those of open thoracotomy,[24] and a prospective, randomized trial of 100 patients who had stage IA NSCLC concluded that long-term survival and local recurrence rates after VATS lobectomy were comparable to those for open thoracotomy.[25] Another study reported a better 5-year survival rate of stage I lung cancer after VATS versus thoracotomy, perhaps due in part to superior postoperative pulmonary function.[26] For the geriatric population, a retrospective study of 32 lobectomy patients 80 years and older (17 VATS, 15 thoracotomy) also demonstrated better 5-year survival following VATS.[27]

To date, most large reports show that across all age groups, VATS lobectomy is safe, with morbidity rates in some reports lower than seen historically with thoracotomy.[24,25,28–31] Other data suggest that pulmonary function as measured by vital capacity and forced expiratory volume in 1 second may be better preserved in patients undergoing VATS rather than thoracotomy.[26] Kirby and colleagues[32] reported that, although they found no difference in intraoperative time, blood loss, or length of hospital stay between patients who underwent VATS versus thoracotomy, the thoracotomy group experienced significantly more postoperative complications, most notably prolonged air leaks. The prospect of superior pulmonary function following VATS relative to thoracotomy has particular significance in the elderly population. Aging alone imparts changes in virtually every aspect of respiratory performance (ie, central regulation, chest wall dynamics, parenchymal elasticity, and gas exchange) and as such, pulmonary complications are a major cause of morbidity and mortality after lung resection in the elderly population (**Box 1**). To determine whether the VATS approach for lobectomy offers specific advantages over thoracotomy in the elderly, retrospective studies have compared the two approaches in aged patient populations. Jaklitsch and colleagues[20] reported that VATS procedures for patients 65 years and older resulted in superior 30-day operative mortality, which was essentially unrelated to age, and a decreased length of hospital stay compared with previous reports for standard thoracotomy. Of the 307 procedures reviewed in this report, however, only 32 involved anatomic resection such as lobectomy or segmentectomy. More recently, Park and colleagues[33] compared data from patients who had undergone elective lobectomy for clinical stage I NSCLC by VATS or thoracotomy and who were in normal sinus rhythm

Box 1
Respiratory changes with aging

Functional manifestations

Increased functional residual capacity

Increased air trapping

Decreased forced expiratory volume exhaled in 1 second

Decreased forced vital capacity

Decreased diffusing capacity

Decreased venous blood oxygenation

Increased closing capacity

Decreased maximal voluntary ventilation

Increased work of breathing

Widened alveolar-arterial gradient for oxygen

Increased dead-space fraction

Increased ventilation-perfusion mismatch

Increased propensity for infection

Decreased resting Pa_{O_2}

Central regulation

Blunted ventilatory response to hypoxia

Blunted ventilatory response to hypercarbia

Increased periodic breathing during sleep

Structural

Decreased number of alveoli

Decreased number of lung capillaries

Decreased elastic recoil, collapse of peripheral airways

Decreased airway size

Decreased alveolar-capillary surface area

Decreased negative intrapleural pressure

Weakening of respiratory muscles

Secretory and immune

Less efficient mucociliary transport

Less sensitive protective airway reflexes

Diminished delayed-type hypersensitivity response to foreign antigens

Increased response to autologous antigens

Decreased polymorphonuclear leukocyte function

Adapted from Castillo MD, Heerdt PM. Pulmonary resection in the elderly. Curr Opin Anaesthesiol 2007;20(1):5; with permission.

preoperatively. Study groups were matched for size (n = 122 in each), age (mean, 67 ± 10 years), sex, comorbidities (chronic obstructive pulmonary disease, hypertension, myocardial infarction, coronary artery disease, diabetes mellitus), and pharmacotherapy (β-blockers and calcium channel blockers). Although the two groups differed in duration of surgery and preoperative pulmonary diffusing capacity, there were no discernable differences with regard to the incidence of individual cardiopulmonary complications (**Table 1**). When all observed postoperative complications were analyzed, however, they occurred with greater frequency in the thoractomy group. To more specifically focus on an advanced-age population, Cattaneo and coauthors[34] analyzed the incidence and grade of postoperative complications in patients 70 years and older undergoing a VATS approach versus a thoracotomy for lobectomy. The two groups were identically matched for age, sex, comorbities, and clinical stage (ie, 90% of each group was stage IA). VATS resulted in a lower overall complication rate, less pulmonary morbidity, and a decreased median length of hospital stay (**Table 2**). In addition, the severity of complications was less in the VATS group, suggesting that the minimally invasive approach can lead to better tolerance in a high-risk, elderly population.

Whether there are cardiovascular benefits to VATS lobectomy remains unclear. Multiple studies have established the relationship between age and the occurrence of atrial fibrillation following lobectomy,[35] with recent data indicating an incidence of 27% in patients older than 60 years when continuous telemetry is used for diagnosis.[36] Two large series have reported lower than expected rates of postoperative atrial fibrillation following VATS lobectomy relative to thoractomy, ranging from 2.9% to 10%.[21,37] These studies, however, did not use routine postoperative telemetry in the highest risk patients (ie, elderly patients) and likely under-reported asymptomatic episodes of atrial fibrillation. In contrast, the matched, case-control study by Park and colleagues[33] comparing 244 patients undergoing lobectomy by VATS or by thoracotomy showed no difference in the rate of postoperative atrial fibrillation, with VATS patients exhibiting a 12% rate of postoperative atrial fibrillation compared with 16% for thoracotomy patients (P = .36). Predictably, in both groups, patients suffering atrial fibrillation were significantly older (median age, 72 years) than those who did not develop the arrhythmia (median age, 66 years).

Changes in cardiac function after lung resection have generally been attributed to an increase in right ventricular (RV) afterload secondary to

Table 1
Comparison of lung resection populations matched for age, sex, comorbidities, and preoperative pharmacotherapy

Data Collected	Thoracotomy (n = 122)	VATS (n = 122)	*P*
Age (years)	67 ± 10	67 ± 10	.99
Surgery duration (hours)	3.0 ± 1.0	3.7 ± 1.0	.001
FEV_1 (% predicted)	86 ± 14	90 ± 19	ns
D_{LCO} (% predicted)	80 ± 18	92 ± 28	.001
Preoperative potassium (mEq/L)	4.4 ± 0.4	4.3 ± 0.4	ns
Preoperative calcium (mg/dL)	9.3 ± 0.6	9.3 ± 0.5	ns
Atelectasis (%)	4.1	1.6	ns
Prolonged air leak (%)	5.7	3.8	ns
Pneumothorax (%)	2.5	0.8	ns
Pneumonitis (%)	4.1	1.6	ns
Atrial fibrillation (%)	16	12	ns
Total complications	27.9	17.2	.05
Deaths	2.5	0	ns

Abbreviations: D_{LCO}, diffusing capacity of lung for carbon monoxide; FEV_1, forced expiratory volume in 1 second; ns, not significant.

Data from Park BJ, Zhang H, Rusch VW, et al. Video-assisted thoracic surgery does not reduce the incidence of postoperative atrial fibrillation after pulmonary lobectomy. J Thorac Cardiovasc Surg 2007;133:775–9.

Table 2
Comparison of lung resection populations older than 70 years and older matched for age, sex, comorbidities, and clinical stage of cancer

Data Collected	Thoracotomy (n = 82)	VATS (n = 82)	*P*
Cardiac disease (%)	45	39	ns
Diabetes mellitus (%)	14	32	.02
% Predicted FEV_1 (median and range)	88 (37–277)	88 (29–136)	ns
% Predicted D_{LCO} (median and range)	83 (36–129)	85 (43–196)	ns
Induction chemotherapy	2	4	ns
Length of stay in days (range)	6 (2–27)	5 (2–20)	< .001
No complications (%)	55	72	.04
Pulmonary	33	15	.01
Atrial fibrillation (%)	23	17	ns
Genitourinary (%)	6	2	ns
Gastrointestinal (%)	5	0	ns
Infectious (%)	5	1	ns
Neurologic (%)	1	4	ns
Death (%)	4	0	ns

Abbreviations: D_{LCO}, diffusing capacity of lung for carbon monixide; FEV_1, forced expiratory volume in 1 second; ns, not significant.

Data from Cattaneo SM, Park BJ, Wilton AS, et al. Use of video-assisted thoracic surgery for lobectomy in the elderly results in fewer complications. Ann Thorac Surg 2008;85(1):231–5.

pulmonary arterial ligation, which ultimately leads to total right heart dilation. Although this simple paradigm is attractive because it potentially accounts for the reduced exercise capacity and enhanced atrial arrhythmogenesis observed after major lung resection by way of thoracotomy, multiple clinical and experimental observations complicate universal application. In particular are data indicating that performance of the right and left ventricles may be depressed following pneumonectomy[38,39] and a study demonstrating that reduced RV ejection fraction following lobectomy is independent of afterload.[40] Given that the cardiovascular sequelae of thoracotomy and lobectomy tend to occur more than 48 hours postoperatively, these studies raise the possibility that a progressive response to overall surgical trauma, not just removal of a segment of the pulmonary circulation, can affect cardiac performance. Accordingly, it has been suggested that in patients who have diminished contractile reserve due to advanced age, cardiac performance in general and RV function in particular may be better preserved by using a minimally invasive surgical technique to perform lobectomy. Nominal support for this contention can be found in a small clinical study of elderly subjects indicating that resting stroke index and RV ejection fraction are significantly higher following lobectomy by way of VATS than by thoracotomy.[41] Potential mechanisms for this response, however, were not explored.

SUMMARY

As the population ages, increasing numbers of elderly patients will present with lung cancer. Due to recent advances in neoadjuvant therapies and accumulating data demonstrating a favorable risk/benefit relationship even in octogenarians, more of these geriatric patients will be surgical candidates. Although preoperative functional status and comorbidities seem to have more of an influence on outcome than age alone, the normal process of cardiopulmonary aging can serve to limit the physiologic reserve necessary to compensate for perioperative stress even in otherwise healthy elderly patients. Emerging experience now also suggests that minimally invasive surgical techniques for the treatment of lung cancer may parallel conventional thoracotomy in terms of oncologic efficacy while decreasing perioperative morbidity in the elderly.

REFERENCES

1. Hurria A, Kris MG. Management of lung cancer in older adults. CA Cancer J Clin 2003;53(6):325–41.

2. Yancik R. Population aging and cancer: a cross-national concern. Cancer J 2005;11(6):437–41.
3. Jemal A, Siegel R, Ward E, et al. Cancer statistics, 2006. CA Cancer J Clin 2006;56(2):106–30.
4. Castillo MD, Heerdt PM. Pulmonary resection in the elderly. Curr Opin Anaesthesiol 2007;20(1):4–9.
5. Ginsberg RJ, Hill LD, Eagan RT, et al. Modern thirty-day operative mortality for surgical resections in lung cancer. J Thorac Cardiovasc Surg 1983;86: 654–8.
6. Wada H, Nakamura T, Nakamoto K, et al. Thirty-day operative mortality for thoracotomy in lung cancer. J Thorac Cardiovasc Surg 1998;115:70–3.
7. Birim O, Zuydendorp HM, Maaat AP, et al. Lung resection for non-small-cell lung cancer in patients older than 70: mortality, morbidity, and late survival compared with the general population. Ann Thorac Surg 2003;76(6):1796–801.
8. Brock MV, Kim MP, Hooker CM, et al. Pulmonary resection in octogenarians with stage I nonsmall cell lung cancer: a 22-year experience. Ann Thorac Surg 2004;77(1):271–7.
9. Pagni S, McKelvey A, Riordan C, et al. Pulmonary resection for malignancy in the elderly: is age still a risk factor? Eur J Cardiothorac Surg 1998;14(1): 40–4 [discussion: 44–5].
10. Hanagiri T, Muranaka H, Hashimoto M, et al. Results of surgical treatment of lung cancer in octogenarians. Lung Cancer 1999;23(2):129–33.
11. Aoki T, Yamato Y, Tsuchida M, et al. Pulmonary complications after surgical treatment of lung cancer in octogenarians. Eur J Cardiothorac Surg 2000;18(6):662–5.
12. Port JL, Kent M, Korst RJ, et al. Surgical resection for lung cancer in the octogenarian. Chest 2004; 126(3):733–8.
13. Matsuoka H, Okada M, Sakamoto T, et al. Complications and outcomes after pulmonary resection for cancer in patients 80 to 89 years of age. Eur J Cardiothorac Surg 2005;28(3):380–3.
14. Watters JM. Surgery in the elderly. Can J Surg 2002; 45(2):104–8.
15. Furuta M, Hayakawa K, Katano S, et al. Radiation therapy for stage I-II non-small cell lung cancer in patients aged 75 years and older. Jpn J Clin Oncol 1996;26:95–8.
16. Wiener DC, Argote-Greene LM, Ramesh H, et al. Choices in the management of asymptomatic lung nodules in the elderly. Surg Oncol 2004;13(4): 239–48.
17. Mery CM, Pappas AN, Bueno R, et al. Similar long-term survival of elderly patients with non-small cell lung cancer treated with lobectomy or wedge resection within the Surveillance, Epidemiology, and End Results database. Chest 2005;128:237–45.
18. Landreneau RJ, Hazelrigg SR, Mack MJ, et al. Postoperative pain-related morbidity: video-assisted thoracic surgery versus thoracotomy. Ann thorac Surg 1993;56(6):1285–9.
19. Sugiura H, Morikawa T, Kaji M, et al. Long-term benefits for the quality of life after video-assisted thorascopic lobectomy in patients with lung cancer. Surg Laparosc Endosc Percutan Tech 1999;9(6): 403–8.
20. Jaklitsch MT, DeCamp MM, Liptay MJ, et al. Video-assisted thoracic surgery in the elderly. A review of 307 cases. Chest 1996;110:751–8.
21. McKenna RJ Jr, Houck W, Fuller CB. Video-assisted thoracic surgery lobectomy: experience with 1,100 cases. Ann Thorac Surg 2006;81(2):421–5 [discussion: 425–6].
22. Yim AP, Landreneau RJ, Izzat MB, et al. Is video-assisted thoracoscopic lobectomy a unified approach? Ann Thorac Surg 1998;66(4):1155–8.
23. Swanson SJ, Herndon JE 2nd, D'Amico TA, et al. Video-assisted thoracic surgery lobectomy: report of CALGB 39802—a prospective, multi-institution feasibility study. J Clin Oncol 2007;25(31):4993–7.
24. Walker WS, Codispoti M, Soon SY, et al. Long-term outcomes following VATS lobectomy for non-small cell bronchogenic carcinoma. Eur J Cardiothorac Surg 2003;23(3):397–402.
25. Sugi K, Kaneda Y, Esato K. Video-assisted thoracoscopic lobectomy achieves a satisfactory long-term prognosis in patients with clinical stage IA lung cancer. World J Surg 2000;24(1):27–30.
26. Kaseda S, Aoki T, Hangai N, et al. Better pulmonary function and prognosis with video-assisted thoracic surgery than with thoracotomy. Ann Thorac Surg 2000;70(5):1644–6.
27. Koizumi K, Haraguchi S, Hirata T, et al. Lobectomy by video-assisted thoracic surgery for lung cancer patients aged 80 years or more. Ann Thorac Cardiovasc Surg 2003;9(1):14–21.
28. Daniels LJ, Balderson SS, Onaitis MW, et al. Thoracoscopic lobectomy: a safe and effective strategy for patients with stage I lung cancer. Ann Thorac Surg 2002;74(3):860–4.
29. Thomas P, Doddoli C, Yena S, et al. VATS is an adequate oncological operation for stage I non-small cell lung cancer. Eur J Cardiothorac Surg 2002;21(6):1094–9.
30. Ohtsuka T, Nomori H, Horio H, et al. Is major pulmonary resection by video-assisted thoracic surgery an adequate procedure in clinical stage I lung cancer? Chest 2004;125(5):1742–6.
31. Gharagozloo F, Tempesta B, Margolis M, et al. Video-assisted thoracic surgery lobectomy for stage I lung cancer. Ann Thorac Surg 2003;76: 10009–15.
32. Kirby TJ, Mack MJ, Landreneau RJ, et al. Lobectomy—video-assisted thoracic surgery versus muscle-sparing thoracotomy: a randomized trial. J Thorac Cardiovasc Surg 1995;109:997–1002.

33. Park BJ, Zhang H, Rusch VW, et al. Video-assisted thoracic surgery does not reduce the incidence of postoperative atrial fibrillation after pulmonary lobectomy. J Thorac Cardiovasc Surg 2007;133: 775–9.
34. Cattaneo SM, Park BJ, Wilton AS, et al. Use of video-assisted thoracic surgery (VATS) for lobectomy in the elderly results in fewer complications. Ann Thorac Surg 2008;85(1):231–5.
35. Amar D. Postthoracotomy atrial fibrillation. Curr Opin Anaesthesiol 2007;20(1):43–7.
36. Amar D, Zhang H, Heerdt PM, et al. Statin use is associated with a reduction in atrial fibrillation after noncardiac thoracic surgery independent of C-reactive protein. Chest 2005;128(5):3421–7.
37. Onaitis MW, Petersen RP, Balderson SS, et al. Thoracoscopic lobectomy is a safe and versatile procedure: experience with 500 consecutive patients. Ann Surg 2006;244(3):420–5.
38. Hsia CCW, Carlin JI, Cassidy SS, et al. Hemodynamic changes after pneumonectomy in the exercising foxhound. J Appl Physiol 1990;69:51–7.
39. Fujisaki T, Gomibuchi M, Shoji T. Changes in left ventricular function during exercise after lung resection—study with a nuclear stethoscope. Nippon Kyobu Geka Gakkai Zasshi 1992;40:1685–92.
40. Reed CE, Dorman BH, Spinale FG. Mechanisms of right ventricular dysfunction after pulmonary resection. Ann Thorac Surg 1996;62:225–31.
41. Mikami I, Koizumi K, Tanaka S. Changes in right ventricular performance in elderly patients who underwent lobectomy using video-assisted thoracic surgery for primary lung cancer. Jpn J Thorac Cardiovasc Surg 2001;49:153–9.

Postoperative Pain Management in the Elderly Undergoing Thoracic Surgery

Marie N. Hanna, MD, Jamie D. Murphy, MD, Kanupriya Kumar, MD, Christopher L. Wu, MD*

KEYWORDS

- Elderly • Pain • Postoperative • Epidural
- Opioid • Nonsteroidal anti-inflammatory agent
- Gabapentin

The management of postoperative pain in the elderly patient undergoing thoracic surgical procedures represents a significant challenge to health care providers. Compared with younger patients, the elderly patient generally is at higher risk for postoperative complications as a result of a variety of factors, including decreased physiologic reserves and increased frequency of comorbidities. Choice of postoperative analgesic regimens may influence perioperative morbidity, particularly in this high-risk group of patients. This article reviews the general considerations for the management of postoperative pain in the elderly patient, the analgesic options available for the treatment of postoperative pain in this group, and the potential risks of these analgesic therapies.

GENERAL CONSIDERATIONS FOR POSTOPERATIVE PAIN MANAGEMENT IN THE ELDERLY

The elderly population, which comprises approximately 12.5% of the total United States population, is expected to increase by 33% during the next few decades and currently accounts for 38% of all health care spending (equivalent to 5% of the United States gross domestic product).[1] Compared with younger patients, the elderly patient generally has decreased physiologic reserves and increased comorbidities (both in frequency and severity), factors that may result in a higher incidence and severity of postoperative complications such as postoperative delirium. Changes that occur in the physiology, pharmacodynamics, pharmacokinetics, and processing of nociceptive information with increasing age may influence the effectiveness of postoperative pain control (**Table 1**). With the elderly patient, there also may be communication, affective, cognitive, social, and ideologic barriers to effective postoperative pain control.

Postoperative pain management in the elderly patient poses several challenges, and these patients may be at higher risk for the undertreatment of severe or uncontrolled postoperative pain. Although clinical studies indicate there is a clinically significant reduction in the intensity of pain perception or symptoms with increasing age,[2] caused in part by a decrease in Aδ and C-fiber nociceptive function and a decrease in sensitivity to low-intensity noxious stimuli,[3,4] these data should not be interpreted as indicating that elderly patients experience less pain than younger patients when they do report the presence of pain. In fact, elderly patients may have an increased response to higher-intensity noxious stimuli and decreased pain tolerance, both of which may contribute to the relatively high incidence of chronic postsurgical pain (CPSP) in elderly patients.[4,5]

Department of Anesthesiology and Critical Care Medicine, The Johns Hopkins University, The Johns Hopkins Hospital, Carnegie 280, 600 North Wolfe Street, Baltimore, MD 21287, USA
* Corresponding author.
E-mail address: chwu@jhmi.edu (C.L. Wu).

Thorac Surg Clin 19 (2009) 353–361
doi:10.1016/j.thorsurg.2009.06.004

thoracic.theclinics.com

Table 1
Physiologic changes in the elderly

System	Changes in Elderly Patients
Anesthetics	↓ Anesthetic requirements for both regional and general anesthesia; ↑duration of action for drugs
Cardiovascular	↑ Incidence of ischemic disease, congestive heart failure, atherosclerotic disease; ↓ cardiac reserve with decreased ability to tolerate perioperative demands
Gastrointestinal	↓ Liver mass and hepatic perfusion; ↓ plasma drug clearance; altered biotransformation and metabolism of drugs secondary to a higher likelihood of polypharmacy treating medical comorbidities
Immune function	↓ Immune responsiveness leading to ↑incidence of perioperative infections
Musculoskeletal/metabolic	↓ Body heat production; ↓ thermoregulatory vasoconstriction; ↓ total body water leading to ↑ peak plasma drug concentrations
Neurological	↑ Incidence of postoperative cognitive dysfunction including ↑ risk for postoperative delirium
Pain	Possible ↓ in intensity of pain perception (experimental) but ↑ response to higher-intensity noxious stimuli; general ↓ in analgesic requirements
Pulmonary	↓ Pulmonary reserve with ↓ vital capacity
Renal	↓ Renal mass, ↓ glomerular filtration rate; ↓ drug excretion

Nevertheless, it is clear that analgesic requirements generally decrease with increasing age. For instance, age has been shown to be the best predictor for both intravenous and neuraxial postoperative morphine requirements.[5] Although both younger and older patients show a large interpatient variability in postoperative analgesic requirements,[5] systemic analgesics generally should be started at a lower dosage inolder patients than in younger patients, in part because of the physiologic and pharmacokinetic effects of aging (eg, longer circulation times, increased sensitivity, and expected longer duration of action resulting from reduced clearance). In elderly patients, a multimodal analgesic approach may be useful by providing analgesia via different mechanisms and, in theory, decreasing the incidence of analgesic-related side effects (because of the decreased dose of each drug received); however, this approach must be used with caution because of the increased risk of adverse drug reactions resulting from polypharmacy in elderly patients.

The presence of affective, cognitive, social, and ideologic barriers may prevent effective postoperative pain management in the elderly patient. Health care providers caring for elderly patients may undertreat pain in this group (relative to younger patients) because of an unfounded level of fear of complications associated with treating perioperative pain. Elderly patients also may contribute to inadequate postoperative pain control, because they may be more reluctant to report pain or take opioid medications. In addition, elderly patients have a higher incidence of affective or cognitive impairments (eg, depression, dementia) that may interfere with effective postoperative pain management.

ANALGESIC OPTIONS

The commonly available analgesic options for elderly patients are similar to those for other patients but must be tailored to account for the pharmacologic and physiologic changes in the elderly patient, including general declines in cardiovascular, respiratory, hepatic, and renal function.[6] Typical options include systemic agents (including opioids and nonsteroidal anti-inflammatory agents [NSAIDS]) and regional analgesic techniques (including epidural, paravertebral, and subcutaneously administered analgesia) generally utilizing local anesthetics or opioids. Although many exotic analgesic agents are available, this discussion is limited to the most commonly used agents.

SYSTEMIC ANALGESIC AGENTS

Opioids

Systemic opioids are among the most common analgesic agents used to treat postoperative pain. Although there may be significant inter-patient differences in the effect of opioids, elderly patients (compared with younger patients) generally have increased central nervous system sensitivity to the effect of opioids and also have decreased clearance and volume of distribution of these agents.[6] Therefore the dosage of opioids should be reduced, regardless of route of administration. Use of intravenous patient-controlled analgesia (IV PCA) in the elderly is appropriate to compensate for the wide inter-patient variability, although postoperative titration of intravenous morphine also can allow successful and safe administration to elderly patients.[7] Age per se is not an impediment to effective postoperative use of IV PCA or patient-controlled epidural analgesia.[8] Some practical guidelines for IV PCA dosing have been published.[9] With regard to patient outcomes after thoracotomy, use of systemic opioids was shown to be statistically inferior to either paravertebral blocks or thoracic epidural analgesia in reducing the risk of postoperative pulmonary complications, although the studies examined were not specifically limited to elderly patients.[10,11] There seems to be no difference between IV PCA and as-needed delivery of opioids with regard to risk of postoperative pulmonary complications (comprising all surgical procedures and patients of all ages).[12]

Nonsteroidal Anti-inflammatory Agents

NSAIDs exert their analgesic effect through the inhibition of peripheral and spinal cyclo-oxygenase (COX) and synthesis of prostaglandins, which may facilitate postoperative pain. There are at least two COX isoforms. COX-1 is constitutive and affects platelet aggregation, hemostasis, and gastric mucosal protection, whereas COX-2 is inducible and is up-regulated with pain, inflammation, and fever. Although NSAIDs generally provide effective analgesia for mild to moderate pain, these agents commonly are used as an adjunct to opioids or regional analgesia for treatment of moderate to severe pain. NSAIDs may be administered orally or parenterally and are particularly useful as components of a multimodal analgesic regimen by producing analgesia through a mechanism different from that of opioids or local anesthetics. For instance, the addition of NSAIDs (including COX-2 inhibitors) IV PCA with opioids results in a statistically significant reduction in postoperative pain scores and significantly decreases morphine consumption with a concurrent reduction in the risk of the opioid-related side effects of nausea, vomiting, and sedation.[13,14,15] For patients specifically undergoing cardiothoracic surgery, the addition of NSAIDs to systemic opioid analgesia reduces the 24-hour visual analogue pain score and opioid requirements, although the use of NSAIDs was not associated with any decrease in mortality or myocardial infarction.[16] Both NSAIDs and acetaminophen have been used to decrease post-thoracotomy ipsilateral shoulder pain.[17,18]

Gabapentin

Gabapentin is an anticonvulsant that originally was designed for the treatment of generalized or partial epileptic seizures; however, it is becoming used more commonly for the treatment of both chronic and acute postoperative pain. Although gabapentin is a structural analogue of the inhibitory neurotransmitter gamma-aminobutyric acid (GABA), it does not bind to GABA receptors.[19] The mechanism of action of gabapentin is not fully understood, although it is likely that gabapentin produces analgesia by binding to and inhibiting the presynaptic voltage-dependent Ca^{2+} channel, decreasing calcium influx and, as a result, inhibiting the release of neurotransmitters (eg, glutamate) from the primary afferent nerve fibers that synapse upon and activate pain-responsive neurons in the spinal cord.[20] A meta-analysis of 12 randomized, controlled trials (RCTs), examining the analgesic efficacy of perioperative gabapentin on patients ($n = 896$) undergoing a variety of surgical procedures found that patients who received gabapentin had significantly lower visual analogue pain scores at 4 hours and 24 hours and less opioid usage; however, gabapentin administration was associated with significantly higher odds of sedation with no difference in the incidence of lightheadedness, dizziness, nausea, or vomiting.[21] Although data from this meta-analysis are not specific for thoracic surgery nor for elderly patients, several more recent individual prospective trials have examined the analgesic efficacy of perioperative gabapentin in patients undergoing thoracic surgery. Two studies noted that gabapentin administered to patients after thoracotomy resulted in a decrease in long-term postthoracotomy pain in patients who underwent video-assisted thoracic surgery, posterolateral/lateral thoracotomy, or median sternotomy.[22,23] An RCT, however, found that preemptively administered gabapentin did not reduce the incidence or severity of postthoracotomy shoulder pain.[24]

REGIONAL ANALGESIA

Epidural Analgesia

Recent (2006) American College of Physicians Guidelines indicate that postoperative pulmonary complications (PPC) continue to be a significant problem.[25] The pathophysiology of pulmonary dysfunction after surgery is multifactorial and may include disruption of normal respiratory muscle activity, spinal reflex inhibition of phrenic nerve activity with subsequent decrease in diaphragmatic function, and uncontrolled postoperative pain leading to splinting.[26] These perioperative pathophysiologies may contribute to hypoventilation, atelectasis, and pneumonia.

The use of perioperative epidural analgesia, particularly in elderly patients who may have decreased physiologic reserves, may be associated with a reduction in the risk for PPCs through provision of superior analgesia and attenuation of perioperative pathophysiologies. Meta-analyses indicate that epidural analgesia (using a local anesthetic-based solution) provides postoperative analgesia superior to that from systemic opioids, including IV PCA.[27,28] The segmental block from thoracic epidural analgesia may result in increased tidal volume and vital capacity related to lower levels of pain and improvement in diaphragmatic activity via interruption of the spinal reflex inhibition of phrenic nerve activity.[29]

Several meta-analyses have examined the effects of epidural analgesia on PPC. The meta-analysis (141 RCTs, n = 9559 patients) compared intraoperative neuraxial (including epidural) anesthesia and general anesthesia. With regard to pulmonary outcomes, the use of neuraxial block (versus general anesthesia) was associated with significantly decreased risk of pneumonia (3.1% vs 6%; odds ratio [OR] = 0.61, 95% confidence interval [CI]: 0.48–0.76), particularly when thoracic epidural was used (OR = 0.48, 95% CI: 0.35–0.67).[30] This finding corroborates an earlier meta-analysis (18 RCTs, n = 1016 patients) that compared various postoperative analgesic techniques and found a reduced risk of PPCs (relative risk [RR] = 0.58, 95% CI: 0.42–0.80) and for pulmonary infections (RR = 0.36, 95% CI: 0.21–0.65) with epidural regimens using local anesthetics.[11] Procedure-specific meta-analyses also have noted a significantly decreased risk of PPC in patients undergoing coronary artery bypass surgery (15 RCTs, n = 644 patients) (17.2% vs 30.3%; OR = 0.41, 95% CI: 0.27–0.60)[31] and also a decreased risk of respiratory failure after open abdominal aortic surgery (6 RCTs, n = 861 patients) (OR = 0.62, 95% CI: 0.51–0.79)[32] with the use of thoracic epidural analgesia.

Although these studies indicate a benefit for epidural analgesia in decreasing the risk of PPC, not all the patients included in these studies were elderly. A 5% random sample of the Medicare claims database from 1997 through 2001 was analyzed for patients undergoing a variety of surgical procedures (colectomy, esophagectomy, gastrectomy, hysterectomy, liver resection, nephrectomy, pulmonary resection, radical retropubic prostatectomy, total knee replacement, Whipple procedure) and was stratified according to the presence (n = 12,780 subjects) or absence (n = 55,943 subjects) for a bill for postoperative epidural analgesia. After adjusting for comorbidities, age, gender, and hospital size, regression analysis revealed that presence of postoperative epidural analgesia was associated with a significantly lower incidence of both 7-day (0.5% vs 0.8%; OR = 0.52, 95% CI: 0.38–0.73) and 30-day (2.1% vs 2.5%; OR = 0.74, 95% CI: 0.63–0.89) mortality.[33] Mortality was significantly lower in patients who received postoperative epidural analgesia for higher-risk procedures (eg, lung resection), but there was no difference in mortality in lower-risk procedures (eg, total knee replacement, hysterectomy) for which patients also had lower comorbidity indices. A separate analysis of Medicare claims only in patients undergoing total hip replacement with and without epidural analgesia also noted a nonsignificant reduction in mortality (0.2% vs 0.4%; OR = 0.6, 95% CI: 0.2–1.5) in this relatively low-risk procedure.[34] In a more specific analysis of the Medicare claims database in patients undergoing lung resection (n = 3501 patients), multivariate regression analysis showed that the presence of epidural analgesia was associated with a significantly lower odds of death at 7 days (OR = 0.39, 95% CI: 0.19–0.80, P = 0.001) and 30 days (OR = 0.53, 95% CI: 0.35–0.78, P = 0.002) after surgery.[35]

Paravertebral Analgesia and Subcutaneous Infusion of Local Anesthetics

Although some analgesic techniques such as epidural analgesia may provide superior analgesia,[27,28] these analgesic modalities may be more labor intensive and expensive than the relatively simple technique of the surgeon directly placing catheters to allow the infusion of local anesthetics into wounds postoperatively. The subcutaneous infusion of local anesthetics is technically easy to place, may be used for several days, and also may be used on an ambulatory basis with portable pumps. There are several mechanisms by which the direct application of local anesthetic to wounds may provide analgesia, including blocking transmission from nociceptive afferents from the wound, inhibiting local inflammatory response to injury which may attenuate pain and hyperalgesia, and possibly suppressing peripheral nociceptor activity via systemic absorption of local anesthetic.

Many RCTs have examined the analgesic effect of subcutaneous infusion of local anesthetics. A meta-analysis of RCTs of subcutaneous continuous wound catheters indicted that this technique resulted in decreased pain scores at rest and with activity (32% reduction, $P < .001$), decreased need for opioids (25% reduction, $P < .001$), decreased risk of nausea and vomiting (16% reduction, $P = .001$), and increased patient satisfaction (30% increase, $P = .007$).[36] No increases in adverse effects were noted. The RCTs for cardiothoracic surgery included 11 trials for thoracotomy primarily for lung resection and two trials for median sternotomy for cardiac surgery. Only continuous infusion and intermittent bolus delivery were studied. For thoracotomy trials, wound catheters were placed in a variety of described peripleural locations (ie, two for extrapleural, two for interpleural, three for intercostal, and four for interpleural sites). For cardiac surgery, one study placed catheters adjacent to the sternum; the other placed subfascial and subcutaneous catheters. Nevertheless, all RCTs reported greater analgesic efficacy (lower pain scores and opioid use) with wound catheters.

RISKS OF AND COMPLICATIONS ASSOCIATED WITH ANALGESIC THERAPIES

Every analgesic modality is associated with risks, although there are differences in the risk profile among these therapies (**Table 2**). The risks and side effects discussed are recognized as general to all postoperative patients and are not specific to thoracic surgery or elderly patients.

Opioids

The use of opioids, regardless of the route of administration, is associated with side effects including postoperative nausea and vomiting, pruritus, urinary retention, and respiratory depression. One of the most feared opioid-related side effects is respiratory depression. With clinically acceptable doses of opioids, the incidence of opioid-related respiratory depression does not seem to differ significantly by route of administration (ie, neuraxial, intravenous, intramuscular, or subcutaneous); the overall incidence is in the range of less than 1%.[37,38] Several factors may be associated with occurrence of respiratory depression, including use of a background infusion (especially in opioid-naïve patients), advanced age, concomitant administration of sedative or hypnotic agents, and coexisting pulmonary disease (eg, sleep apnea).[37,38] Guidelines for the perioperative management of patients who have obstructive sleep apnea indicate that in these patients the use of opioids should be avoided when possible.[39]

Nonsteroidal Anti-inflammatory Agents

Perioperative administration of NSAIDs may be associated with several complications (eg, decreased hemostasis [platelet], renal dysfunction, and gastrointestinal hemorrhage) that result from the inhibition of COX and prostaglandins formation. Although decreased hemostasis from NSAID use is attributed to platelet dysfunction resulting from inhibition of thromboxane A_2 (an important mediator of platelet aggregation and vasoconstriction),[40] the evidence of the effect of NSAIDs on postoperative bleeding in general is uncertain, because a surveillance study of perioperative ketorolac did not demonstrate a significant increase in operative site bleeding.[41] Perioperative NSAID-induced renal dysfunction is uncommon in euvolemic patients who have normal renal function but may occur in high-risk patients (eg, those who have hypovolemia, abnormal renal function, or abnormal serum electrolytes), because prostaglandins may dilate renal vascular beds.[42] A higher incidence of gastrointestinal bleeding may be associated with perioperative use of NSAIDs because of the inhibition of cytoprotective gastric mucosal prostaglandins, although a meta-analysis found no increased risk of gastrointestinal bleeding.[16,41] COX-2 inhibitors are associated with a lower incidence of gastrointestinal complications[43] and exhibit minimal platelet inhibition even when administered in supratherapeutic doses,[44] but the long-term use of COX-2 inhibitors has been associated with excess cardiovascular risk.[45] The perioperative safety of COX-2 inhibitors is essentially uncertain; however, use of COX-2 inhibitors may be associated with increased incidence of cardiovascular events after coronary artery bypass graft surgery.[46,47,48]

Regional Analgesic Techniques

Despite the potential benefits of regional techniques for perioperative anesthesia and analgesia, there are several risks associated with these techniques. Common medication-related (ie, local anesthetic, opioids) side effects for epidural analgesia include nausea and vomiting, pruritus, hypotension, motor block, and, less commonly, respiratory depression. Nausea and vomiting associated with a single administration of neuraxial opioid (typically morphine) occurs in

Table 2
Benefits and risks of common analgesic regimens

Therapeutic Regimen	Advantages	Disadvantages
Systemic opioids	No analgesic ceiling Many possible routes of administration	Nausea, vomiting, pruritis, urinary retention, sedation Increased risk of respiratory depression Development of tolerance and physical dependence Caution in patients who have obstructive sleep apnea
Nonsteroidal anti-inflammatory agents	Generally nonsedating Opioid-sparing effect Non-addictive	Increased risk of bleeding (secondary to platelet dysfunction) Gastrointestinal distress (including ulceration and hemorrhage) Caution with renal insufficiency
Gabapentin	Opioid-sparing effect Non-addictive ? Decrease in chronic postsurgical pain	Sedation
Epidural analgesia	↓ Postoperative pulmonary complications Superior analgesia (versus opioids)	Hypotension, motor block, inadvertent spinal anesthesia Technique is more invasive than systemic opioids Caution with anticoagulants (low molecular weight heparin)
Paravertebral analgesia	↓ Postoperative pulmonary complications Unilateral block, hemodynamic stability Superior analgesia (versus opioids)	Accidental epidural or intrathecal injection Technique is more invasive than systemic opioids

approximately 20% to 50% of patients.[49] The overall incidence of pruritus associated with neuraxial opioids is approximately 60% but is lower (approximately 15%) with epidural local anesthetics.[50] The incidence of postoperative hypotension with postoperative epidural analgesia has been reported to be approximately 0.7% to 3%, although the incidence of clinically relevant hypotension is uncertain.[51,52] The use of local anesthetics for postoperative epidural analgesia may contribute to lower extremity motor block in 2% to 3% of patients,[51,52] but this side effect is less common with thoracic epidurals. The incidence of respiratory depression associated with neuraxial administration of opioids is dose dependent and is approximately 0.1% to 0.9%; it should be noted, however, that the incidence of respiratory depression with neuraxial opioids (when used in appropriate doses) is not higher than that seen with systemic administration of opioids.[38,53]

Neurologic injury is a potentially devastating but uncommon complication from regional analgesic techniques; a recent systemic review of 32 studies revealed that the rate of permanent neurologic injury after spinal and epidural anesthesia ranged from 0 to 4.2:10,000 and from 0 to7.6:10,000, respectively.[54] During the past 10 to 15 years, a significant concern with combination of postoperative epidural analgesia and more potent anticoagulants (particularly the newer low molecular weight heparins) has been the potential for the development of epidural hematoma and permanent paralysis. Although a detailed discussion is beyond the scope of this article, it is clear that different types and classes of anticoagulants have different pharmacokinetic properties that affect the timing of both neuraxial catheter/needle insertion and catheter removal. The American Society of Regional Anesthesia and Pain Medicine has published a series of consensus statements regarding the concurrent use of anticoagulants and neuraxial techniques.[55] Infection-related complications may occur in association with continuous regional analgesia catheters. For epidural catheters, the incidence of epidural abscesses has been reported to be less than 0.1%; in one series, no patient who had an epidural catheter in situ for fewer than 3 days developed an epidural abscess, and eight of the nine patients who developed an epidural abscess were classified as immunocompromised.[56,57]

Chronic Postsurgical Pain

CPSP can be extremely debilitating and may occur in 22% to 67% of patients undergoing thoracotomy, with a significant percentage of these patients experiencing severe CPSP.[58] Many predictive factors have been identified for the development of CPSP, including the presence of moderate to severe acute postoperative pain.[59] Although it would seem reasonable that an intervention that could decrease the severity of acute postoperative pain would decrease the incidence or severity of CPSP, a causal relationship between the severity of acute postoperative pain and the incidence or severity of CPSP has not been established definitively. Despite this uncertainty, a number of studies examining the administration of a variety of analgesic interventions in an attempt to attenuate the incidence or severity of CPSP suggest that use of epidural analgesia[60,61,62] or other systemic agents[63,64,65] may be associated with a decrease in the incidence or severity of CPSP.

SUMMARY

The management of postoperative pain in the elderly represents a considerable challenge because these patients are generally at higher risk for postoperative complications. There are several analgesic options, some of which may influence perioperative morbidity in this high-risk group of patients. Although use of regional analgesia, particularly epidural analgesia is associated with some benefits,[65,66] including a decrease in perioperative morbidity,[29] there are side effects and complications (eg, medication-related side effects, epidural hematoma, infection)[67,68,69,70] from these and other techniques, and the clinician should evaluate the benefits and risks of each technique on an individual basis.[71] Nevertheless, the available data suggest that use of regional analgesic techniques (ie, epidural and paravertebral catheters) is associated with a decrease in perioperative pulmonary complications.

REFERENCES

1. Anderson GF, Hussey PS. Population aging: a comparison among industrialized countries. Health Aff 2000;19:191–203.
2. Gibson SJ, Helme RD. Age-related differences in pain perception and report. Clin Geriatr Med 2001; 17:433–56.
3. Gregoratos G. Clinical manifestations of acute myocardial infarction in older patients. Am J Geriatr Cardiol 1998;7:35–40.
4. Gloth FM 3rd. Geriatric pain. Factors that limit pain relief and increase complications. Geriatrics 2000; 55:46–54.
5. Macintyre PE, Jarvis DA. Age is the best predictor of postoperative morphine requirements. Pain 1996;64: 357–64.
6. Aubrun F. Management of postoperative analgesia in elderly patients. Reg Anesth Pain Med 2005;30: 363–79.
7. Aubrun F, Monsel S, Langeron O, et al. Postoperative titration of intravenous morphine in the elderly patient. Anesthesiology 2002;96:17–23.
8. Gagliese L, Jackson M, Ritvo P, et al. Age is not an impediment to effective use of patient-controlled analgesia by surgical patients. Anesthesiology 2000;93:601–10.
9. Lavand'Homme P, De Kock M. Practical guidelines on the postoperative use of patient-controlled analgesia in the elderly. Drugs Aging 1998;13:9–16.
10. Joshi GP, Bonnet F, Shah R, et al. A systematic review of randomized trials evaluating regional techniques for postthoracotomy analgesia. Anesth Analg 2008;107:1026–40.
11. Ballantyne JC, Carr DB, deFerranti S, et al. The comparative effects of postoperative analgesic therapies on pulmonary outcome: cumulative meta-analyses of randomized, controlled trials. Anesth Analg 1998;86:598–612.
12. Hudcova J, McNicol E, Quah C, et al. Patient controlled opioid analgesia versus conventional opioid analgesia for postoperative pain. Cochrane Database Syst Rev 2006;(4):CD003348.
13. Elia N, Lysakowski C, Tramer MR. Does multimodal analgesia with acetaminophen, nonsteroidal antiinflammatory drugs, or selective cyclooxygenase-2 inhibitors and patient-controlled analgesia morphine offer advantages over morphine alone? Meta-analyses of randomized trials. Anesthesiology 2005; 103:1296–304.
14. Straube S, Derry S, McQuay HJ, et al. Effect of preoperative Cox-II-selective NSAIDs (coxibs) on postoperative outcomes: a systematic review of randomized studies. Acta Anaesthesiol Scand 2005;49:601–13.
15. Marret E, Kurdi O, Zufferey P, et al. Effects of nonsteroidal antiinflammatory drugs on patient-controlled

analgesia morphine side effects: meta-analysis of randomized controlled trials. Anesthesiology 2005; 102:1249–60.

16. Bainbridge D, Cheng DC, Martin JE, et al. NSAID-analgesia, pain control and morbidity in cardiothoracic surgery. Can J Anaesth 2006;53:46–59.
17. Mac TB, Girard F, Chouinard P, et al. Acetaminophen decreases early post-thoracotomy ipsilateral shoulder pain in patients with thoracic epidural analgesia: a double-blind placebo-controlled study. J Cardiothorac Vasc Anesth 2005;19:475–8.
18. Singh H, Bossard RF, White PF, et al. Effects of ketorolac versus bupivacaine coadministration during patient-controlled hydromorphone epidural analgesia after thoracotomy procedures. Anesth Analg 1997;84:564–9.
19. Taylor CP, Gee NS, Su T, et al. A summary of the mechanistic hypotheses of gabapentin pharmacology. Epilepsy Res 1998;29:233–49.
20. Shimoyama M, Shimoyama N, Hori Y. Gabapentin affects glutamatergic excitatory neurotransmission in the rat dorsal horn. Pain 2000;85:405–14.
21. Hurley RW, Cohen SM, Williams KA, et al. The efficacy of perioperative oral gabapentin on postoperative recovery. Reg Anesth Pain Med 2006;31:237–47.
22. Sihoe AD, Lee TW, Wan IY, et al. The use of gabapentin for post-operative and post-traumatic pain in thoracic surgery patients. Eur J Cardiothorac Surg 2006;29:795–9.
23. Solak O, Metin M, Esme H, et al. Effectiveness of gabapentin in the treatment of chronic post-thoracotomy pain. Eur J Cardiothorac Surg 2007;32:9–12.
24. Huot MP, Chouinard P, Girard F, et al. Gabapentin does not reduce post-thoracotomy shoulder pain: a randomized, double-blind placebo-controlled study. Can J Anaesth 2008;55:337–43.
25. Qaseem A, Snow V, Fitterman N, et al. Risk assessment for and strategies to reduce perioperative pulmonary complications for patients undergoing noncardiothoracic surgery: a guideline from the American College of Physicians. Ann Intern Med 2006;144:575–80.
26. Warner DO. Preventing postoperative pulmonary complications: the role of the anesthesiologist. Anesthesiology 2000;92:1467–72.
27. Block BM, Liu SS, Rowlingson AJ, et al. Efficacy of postoperative epidural analgesia: a meta-analysis. JAMA 2003;290:2455–63.
28. Wu CL, Cohen SR, Richman JM, et al. Efficacy of postoperative patient-controlled and continuous infusion epidural analgesia versus intravenous patient-controlled analgesia with opioids: a meta-analysis. Anesthesiology 2005;103:1079–88.
29. Liu SS, Wu CL. Effect of postoperative analgesia on major postoperative complications: a systematic update of the evidence. Anesth Analg 2007;104: 689–702.
30. Rodgers A, Walker N, Schug S, et al. Reduction of postoperative mortality and morbidity with epidural or spinal anaesthesia: results from overview of randomised trials. BMJ 2000;321:1493.
31. Liu SS, Block BM, Wu CL. Effects of perioperative central neuraxial analgesia on outcome after coronary artery bypass surgery: a meta-analysis. Anesthesiology 2004;101:153–61.
32. Nishimori M, Ballantyne JC, Low JHS. Epidural pain relief versus systemic opioid based pain relief for abdominal aortic surgery. Cochrane Database Syst Rev 2006;(3):CD005059.
33. Wu CL, Hurley RW, Anderson GF, et al. The effect of perioperative epidural analgesia on patient mortality and morbidity in the Medicare population. Reg Anesth Pain Med 2004;29:525–33.
34. Wu CL, Anderson GF, Herbert R, et al. The effect of perioperative epidural analgesia on patient mortality and morbidity in the Medicare population undergoing total hip replacement. Reg Anesth Pain Med 2003;28:271–8.
35. Wu CL, Saperstein A, Herbert R, et al. Effect of perioperative epidural analgesia on patient mortality and morbidity in the Medicare population undergoing partial lobectomy. J Clin Anesth 2006; 18:515–20.
36. Liu SS, Richman JM, Thirlby RC, et al. Efficacy of continuous wound catheters delivering local anesthetic for postoperative analgesia: a quantitative and qualitative systematic review of randomized controlled trials. J Am Coll Surg 2006;203: 914–32.
37. Looi-Lyons LC, Chung FF, Chan VW, et al. Respiratory depression: an adverse outcome during patient-controlled analgesia therapy. J Clin Anesth 1996;8:151–6.
38. Etches RC. Respiratory depression associated with patient-controlled analgesia: a review of eight cases. Can J Anaesth 1994;41:125–32.
39. Gross JB, Bachenberg KL, Benumof JL, et al. Practice guidelines for the perioperative management of patients with obstructive sleep apnea: a report by the American Society of Anesthesiologists Task Force on Perioperative Management of patients with obstructive sleep apnea. Anesthesiology 2006;104:1081–93.
40. Fitzgerald GA. Cardiovascular pharmacology of nonselective nonsteroidal anti-inflammatory drugs and coxibs: clinical considerations. Am J Cardiol 2002;89:26D–32D.
41. Strom BL, Berlin JA, Kinman JL, et al. Parenteral ketorolac and risk of gastrointestinal and operative site bleeding. A postmarketing surveillance study. JAMA 1996;275:376–82.
42. Whelton A. Nephrotoxicity of nonsteroidal antiinflammatory drugs: physiologic foundations and clinical implications. Am J Med 1999;106:13S–24S.

43. Laine L. Gastrointestinal safety of coxibs and outcomes studies: what's the verdict? J Pain Symptom Manage 2002;23(Suppl 2):S5–14.
44. Leese PT, Hubbard RC, Karim A, et al. Effects of celecoxib, a novel cyclooxygenase-2 inhibitor, on platelet function in healthy adults: a randomized, controlled trial. J Clin Pharmacol 2000;40:124–32.
45. Brophy JM. Celecoxib and cardiovascular risks. Expert Opin Drug Saf 2005;4:1005–15.
46. Kharasch ED. Perioperative COX-2 inhibitors: knowledge and challenges. Anesth Analg 2004;98:1–3.
47. Nussmeier NA, Whelton AA, Brown MT, et al. Safety and efficacy of the cyclooxygenase-2 inhibitors parecoxib and valdecoxib after noncardiac surgery. Anesthesiology 2006;104:518–26.
48. Nussmeier NA, Whelton AA, Brown MT, et al. Complications of the COX-2 inhibitors parecoxib and valdecoxib after cardiac surgery. N Engl J Med 2005;352:1081–91.
49. Chaney MA. Side effects of intrathecal and epidural opioids. Can J Anaesth 1995;42:891–903.
50. Kjellberg F, Tramer MR. Pharmacological control of opioid-induced pruritus: a quantitative systematic review of randomized trials. Eur J Anaesthesiol 2001;18:346–57.
51. Wheatley RG, Schug SA, Watson D. Safety and efficacy of postoperative epidural analgesia. Br J Anaesth 2001;87:47–61.
52. Liu SS, Allen HW, Olsson GL. Patient-controlled epidural analgesia with bupivacaine and fentanyl on hospital wards: prospective experience with 1,030 surgical patients. Anesthesiology 1998;88:688–95.
53. de Leon-Casasola OA, Parker BM, Lema MJ, et al. Epidural analgesia versus intravenous patient-controlled analgesia. Differences in the postoperative course of cancer patients. Reg Anesth 1994;19:307–15.
54. Brull R, McCartney CJ, Chan VW, et al. Neurological complications after regional anesthesia: contemporary estimates of risk. Anesth Analg 2007;104:965–74.
55. Horlocker TT, Wedel DJ, Benzon H, et al. Regional anesthesia in the anticoagulated patient: defining the risks (the second ASRA Consensus Conference on Neuraxial Anesthesia and Anticoagulation). Reg Anesth Pain Med 2003;28:172–97.
56. Cameron CM, Scott DA, McDonald WM, et al. A review of neuraxial epidural morbidity: experience of more than 8,000 cases at a single teaching hospital. Anesthesiology 2007;106:997–1002.
57. Wang LP, Hauerberg J, Schmidt JF. Incidence of spinal epidural abscess after epidural analgesia: a national 1-year survey. Anesthesiology 1999;91:1928–36.
58. Kehlet H, Jensen TS, Woolf CJ. Persistent postsurgical pain: risk factors and prevention. Lancet 2006;367:1618–25.
59. Perkins FM, Kehlet H. Chronic pain as an outcome of surgery. A review of predictive factors. Anesthesiology 2000;93:1123–33.
60. Lavand'homme P, De Kock M, Waterloos H. Intraoperative epidural analgesia combined with ketamine provides effective preventive analgesia in patients undergoing major digestive surgery. Anesthesiology 2005;103:813–20.
61. Senturk M, Ozcan PE, Talu GK, et al. The effects of three different analgesia techniques on long-term postthoracotomy pain. Anesth Analg 2002;94:11–5.
62. Obata H, Saito S, Fujita N, et al. Epidural block with mepivacaine before surgery reduces long-term post-thoracotomy pain. Can J Anaesth 1999;46:1127–32.
63. Reuben SS, Ekman EF, Raghunathan K, et al. The effect of cyclooxygenase-2 inhibition on acute and chronic donor-site pain after spinal-fusion surgery. Reg Anesth Pain Med 2006;31:6–13.
64. Reuben SS, Makari-Judson G, Lurie SD. Evaluation of efficacy of the perioperative administration of venlafaxine XR in the prevention of postmastectomy pain syndrome. J Pain Symptom Manage 2004;27:133–9.
65. Rathmell JP, Wu CL, Sinatra RS, et al. Acute post-surgical pain management: a critical appraisal of current practice, December 2–4, 2005. Reg Anesth Pain Med 2006;31(4 Suppl 1):1–42.
66. Liu SS, Wu CL. The effect of analgesic technique on postoperative patient-reported outcomes including analgesia: a systematic review. Anesth Analg 2007;105:789–808.
67. Hebl JR. The importance and implications of aseptic techniques during regional anesthesia. Reg Anesth Pain Med 2006;31:311–23.
68. Wedel DJ, Horlocker TT. Regional anesthesia in the febrile or infected patient. Reg Anesth Pain Med 2006;31:324–33.
69. Horlocker TT, Wedel DJ. Regional anesthesia in the immunocompromised patient. Reg Anesth Pain Med 2006;31:334–45.
70. Porterfield WR, Wu CL. Epidural hematoma in an ambulatory surgical patient. J Clin Anesth 1997;9:74–7.
71. Bergqvist D, Wu CL, Neal JM. Anticoagulation and neuraxial regional anesthesia: perspectives. Reg Anesth Pain Med 2003;28:163–6.

Evaluation and Management of the Elderly Patient at Risk for Postoperative Delirium

Anita S. Bagri, MD[a,*], Alex Rico, MD[b], Jorge G. Ruiz, MD[b,c]

KEYWORDS

• Confusion • Surgery • Perioperative care • Geriatrics

Delirium is a common complication afflicting post-surgical geriatric patients. It is a medical emergency characterized by the acute onset of changes in cognition or attention that fluctuate throughout the course of a day. Up to 40% of hospitalized elderly patients experience delirium;[1] postoperatively, the incidence varies according to the type of surgery. The consequences of delirium can be devastating and impact mortality and morbidity in the medical, functional, psychological, and social domains.[2–15] Additionally, the economic burden of delirium is enormous. The treatment of delirium cost Medicare $6.9 billion in 2004 alone.[16] Those who experience delirium during hospitalization are more likely to use twice as many health care dollars in the following year, increasing the estimated total annual cost of delirium to $38 to $152 billion.[17] Thus, prevention, timely recognition, and targeted treatment may reduce the incidence of delirium and decrease the cost of postsurgical care. The purpose of this review is to summarize the findings in the literature concerning risk factors, preventive measures, diagnostic and screening instruments, and management strategies for postoperative delirium and to offer recommendations to the clinician caring for elderly surgical patients.

PATHOGENESIS

The underlying mechanisms contributing to delirium are poorly understood. Many theories emphasize aberrant neurotransmission. One of the most widely accepted mechanisms is cholinergic deficiency; increased serum anticholinergic activity is associated with delirium.[18] Other hypotheses invoke abnormalities in melatonin and serotonin,[19,20] with abnormal tryptophan metabolism unifying these ideas because tryptophan is a precursor for both.[21] Noradrenergic hyperactivity has also been implicated.[22]

Neuronal damage is an alternative explanation, secondary either to oxidative stress [23] or inflammation. Proinflammatory cytokines increase in postoperative delirium,[24] especially interleukin-6 and interleukin-8.[25] In addition, elevations in C-reactive protein occur in delirious patients.[9] A link between inflammation and neurotransmission has been proposed, with inflammation-induced perivascular edema leading to hypoxia and subsequent reduced synthesis of acetylcholine.[26]

It is generally thought that delirium represents global brain dysfunction. Electroencephalographic findings reveal a decrease in the fast alpha frequencies and an increase in the slower theta rhythm.[27] In hypoactive delirium, hypoperfusion

A version of this article originally appeared in the November 2008 issue of Clinics in Geriatric Medicine

[a] Geriatric Research, Education and Clinical Center (11GRC), Bruce W. Carter Veterans Affairs Medical Center, 1201 NW 16 Street, Miami, FL 33125, USA
[b] University of Miami Miller School of Medicine, P.O. Box 016960 (R-100), Miami, Florida 33101, USA
[c] Stein Gerontological Institute, Miami Jewish Home and Hospital, 5200 NE 2 Avenue, Miami, FL 33137, USA
* Corresponding author.
E-mail address: anita.bagri@va.gov (A.S. Bagri).

Thorac Surg Clin 19 (2009) 363–376
doi:10.1016/j.thorsurg.2009.06.005
1547-4127/09/$ – see front matter

occurs globally in the frontal, temporal, and occipital lobes, and focally in the caudate head, thalamus, and lenticular nuclei. Delirium improves once blood flow returns to normal, suggesting that cerebral hypoperfusion may play a role.[28]

RISK FACTORS

Inouye[29–31] categorized risk factors for postoperative delirium into predisposing factors inherent to the patient that increase baseline vulnerability and precipitating factors, which are the conditions during the perioperative period that trigger the development of delirium (**Table 1**). The interaction of these factors remains complex.[29–31]

PREDISPOSING RISK FACTORS

Various cohort and randomized studies consistently demonstrate the relationship of older age to increasing incidence of delirium.[3,7,9,14,32–43] Homeostenosis, the reduction in physiologic reserve with age, offers one possible explanation.[44] There is no consensus regarding the effect of gender, with some studies reporting a higher risk for women,[36,43,45] others for men,[3,4,46,47] but the majority revealing no gender predilection.[7,14,32,38–40,48,49] Vision or hearing impairment is consistently associated with greater risk.[9,12,38,41]

Impaired cognitive function contributes to delirium risk. Dementia and low scores on the Folstein Mini-Mental State Examination (MMSE) confer higher risk for postoperative delirium.[4,8,9,11,12,35,37–39,41,42,50–53] Abnormal performance on the clock-drawing test also increases risk,[47] which lends support to the hypothesis that impairments in executive function, rather than memory deficits, are more important indicators.[54] Slower reaction times on neuropsychiatric tests are also associated with delirium,

Table 1
Risk factors for the development of postoperative delirium

Predisposing	Precipitating
Widely accepted factors	
1. Age[3,7,9,14,32–43] 2. Cognitive impairment[4,8,9,11,12,35,37–39,41,42,50–53] 3. Lower education level[38,43,48,56] 4. Sensory impairment[9,12,38,41] 5. Decreased functional status[8,33,36,37,42,43] 6. Comorbid medical illness[3,7,9,10,32,36,40,49,52,57] 7. Malnutrition[31,39,58] 8. Depression[8,9,38,41,43,59]	1. Orthopedic > vascular > cardiac[10,32,39,52,57,64,65] 2. Urgent or emergent procedure[7,10,70] 3. Delayed surgery after hip fracture[11] 4. Preoperative hemodynamic instability[7,10] 5. Hypoxemia[59,62] 6. Electrolyte disturbance[9,37,38,40,42,49] 7. Transfusion requirement[7,9,10,72] 8. Sleep deprivation[40] 9. Urinary catheter[31] 10. Immobility[75] 11. Poorly controlled pain[35,36,43] 12. Polypharmacy[31] Benzodiazepines[18,33,42,50,78] Anticholinergics[59,79–81] 13. Meperidine[36,78,82]
Controversial factors	
1. History of delirium[42] 2. Gender Female[36,43,45] Male[3,4,46,47] No association[7,14,32,38–40,48,49] 3. Alcohol use or abuse[34,35,37] 4. Tobacco use[3,9,50] 5. Apolipoprotein E ϵ4 carrier status[63]	1. Longer operations[7,10,39,40]
Factors with no effect	
1. Preoperative anxiety[61,62]	1. General versus regional anesthesia[43,48,59,72] 2. Route of postoperative analgesia[34,35,67,72,76] 3. Type of opioid (except meperidine)[78,82,84–86]

suggesting that preexisting deficits in attention contribute to risk.[55] In one study, subjective memory complaints in patients older than 60 years undergoing cardiac surgery conferred a threefold higher risk for developing delirium postoperatively.[52]

Lower education level increases delirium risk,[38,43,48,56] and when present, delirium is of longer duration.[50] The cognitive reserve theory is often cited to explain this finding.[56] In fact, one study estimates that those who complete seventh grade are at a 60% higher risk for delirium when compared with those who complete high school.[56]

Poor functional status is associated with delirium.[8,36,37,42] Requiring assistance with one or more activities of daily living (ADLs) confers a 54% increased risk.[33] Patients admitted from nursing homes, implying self-care deficits, are more likely to develop postoperative delirium than their community-dwelling counterparts.[12,38] Dependence in instrumental ADLs also augments risk.[43]

Other comorbid medical diseases increase the likelihood of developing postoperative delirium. Diabetes, stroke, peripheral vascular disease, atrial fibrillation, heart failure, anemia, and prior or perioperative myocardial infarction increase the probability of postoperative delirium according to some studies, but these are not consistently associated.[3,7,9,10,32,36,40,49,52,57] Poor nutritional status increases the risk for delirium fourfold.[31,39,58] A higher number of comorbidities[57] and higher severity of illness based on Acute Physiology and Chronic Health Evaluation, version 2 (APACHE II) score[41] also predict greater risk.

Prior psychiatric disease may augment delirium risk. A history of delirium is reported to increase risk,[42] although other studies refute this association.[9] Preexisting depression and higher number of depressive symptoms on the Geriatric Depression Scale are associated with postoperative delirium[8,9,41,43,59] and longer duration of episodes,[50,60] with 1 study reporting a threefold increase in risk.[38] No relationship between preoperative anxiety and postoperative delirium has been shown.[61,62]

Social and lifestyle factors may also exert an effect on the development of postoperative delirium. Some studies,[34,35,37] but not all,[9,14,38,43,49,62] have reported that alcohol use or abuse increases risk for delirium. Past or present tobacco use increases risk,[3,9] with the number of pack-years smoked being the most important factor.[50] Again, this association is not consistently demonstrated.[7,49,57] Marital status may also play a role; those who are single, widowed, separated, or divorced are at a higher risk.[50]

There is limited evidence to suggest that genetics may play a role in the development of postoperative delirium. In 1 study, apolipoprotein E ϵ4 carrier status conferred an almost fourfold higher risk after adjusting for covariates, such as age, education, and functional status.[63] However, another study found no effect.[45] It remains to be determined if this association occurs independent of dementia.

PRECIPITATING RISK FACTORS

The type of surgery affects the delirium rates. The incidence is highest after orthopedic procedures, with a range of 16% to 62% after femoral neck fracture repairs.[64] Estimates for delirium after vascular surgery are 29.1% to 42.3%.[39,65] The incidence of postoperative delirium after cardiac surgery is 8.4% to 41.7%.[10,32,52,57] Specifically, risk with valve surgery is greater than with coronary artery bypass grafting surgery,[10] almost fourfold higher according to one study.[52] After general surgery, delirium occurs 7% of the time,[66] but estimates increase to 26% after major abdominal surgery for cancer (mainly colectomy).[67] Data on the incidence of delirium after laparoscopic surgery are scarce. In contrast to the more invasive surgeries mentioned earlier, delirium after cataract surgery occurs less than 5% of the time.[68,69]

Emergency surgery, as opposed to elective surgery, may also increase delirium risk. A meta-analysis of 26 studies found a 16.2% increase in absolute risk for delirium in hip fracture patients compared with patients undergoing elective orthopedic procedures,[70] with 1 study implicating greater pain in the fracture group as a possible explanation.[14] Longer waiting times for operations after hip fracture may also increase risk.[11] Urgent or emergent cardiac operations, compared with elective surgery, are associated with higher incidence of delirium postoperatively,[7,10] but no difference was seen when urgent and elective thoracic surgeries were compared.[40] Agnoletti and colleagues[71] are currently conducting a study to investigate further the effect of elective versus emergency surgery on postoperative delirium.

There is no consensus on the effect of intraoperative factors on delirium risk. Some studies report no association between total surgery duration and delirium,[9,32,46,50,62] whereas others demonstrate higher risk after longer operations.[7,10,39,40] There is no difference in delirium rates for those receiving general versus regional anesthesia.[43,48,59,72] Comparisons among various anesthetic agents also reveal similar incidence.[33,73] Intraoperative hypotension may be a risk factor for delirium,[13] but again, this is not consistently identified.[9,72] Hemodynamic instability or requiring an intra-aortic balloon pump increases the risk for delirium after cardiac surgery by as much as 24%.[7,10]

Immediate postoperative events, such as hypoxemia,[59,62] dehydration,[74] and disturbances of sodium, potassium, and glucose increase the risk for developing delirium.[9,37,38,40,42,49] Postoperative RBC transfusion requirement, especially for a hematocrit value of less than 30%, may augment risk,[7,9,10,72] although some studies do not show any relationship.[40] Sleep deprivation increases the likelihood,[40] as does the presence of a urinary catheter.[31] Each day of delayed ambulation after hip surgery confers a 72% increased risk for delirium.[75] There are no data on the effect of postoperative hypotension and delirium risk.

Poorly controlled postoperative pain is a risk factor for delirium.[35,43] Patients with severe pain are 9 times as likely to develop delirium.[36] Interestingly, higher pain scores at rest are predictive compared with those for pain with movement or maximal pain.[35,36] Comparisons among epidural, intravenous, intrathecal, and oral postoperative analgesia show no difference in delirium rates.[34,35,67,72,76] However, oral agents may reduce likelihood,[43,77] with 1 study estimating a fourfold reduction with oral opioids versus intravenous patient-controlled analgesia opioids.[33]

Polypharmacy is a risk factor for delirium, as are certain classes of medications. Drug toxicity accounts for up to 40% of delirium in medical and surgical patients.[1] Starting more than 3 new medications increases risk by almost threefold.[31] Preoperative, perioperative, and postoperative use of benzodiazepines augments risk by almost threefold.[18,33,42,50,78] Anticholinergic medications are hazardous,[59,79,80] especially diphenhydramine.[81] Some data suggest that preoperative antidepressant use and antipsychotics also increase risk.[18,42,50] Preoperative chronic use of opioids is associated with delirium,[42] although in this case, delirium may be a surrogate for pain severity.

Among opioids, only meperidine increases risk for delirium,[36,78,82] probably because its metabolite normeperidine has anticholinergic and stimulant activity in the central nervous system. However, none of these cohort studies comments on the efficacy of analgesia, which may play an important role.[83] Morphine, fentanyl, hydromorphone, tramadol, oxycodone, and codeine are all associated with similar rates of delirium.[78,82,84–86]

PREVENTION

Delirium is an adverse outcome and often an indicator of the quality of health care.[87] Moreover, as much as 50% of the delirium in medical and surgical patients can be prevented.[87] Modification of known risk factors remains the cornerstone of all strategies.

The data are scarce regarding interventions related to the surgery itself. Beating-heart cardiac surgery (off-pump) may lower the incidence of delirium when compared with conventional cardiopulmonary bypass, but the off-pump group in this nonrandomized study had more favorable baseline characteristics, which may have decreased their likelihood for developing delirium.[10]

Given that there are usually several risk factors present, it logically follows that most interventions are multimodal. Rarely is one intervention implemented alone. Inouye and colleagues[88] intervened on 6 risk factors in geriatric medical patients (cognitive impairment, sleep deprivation, immobility, dehydration, visual impairment, and hearing impairment) and showed an absolute risk reduction in delirium of 6.1% compared with usual care. Frequent orientation, sleep hygiene, early mobilization, visual aids and large-print books, hearing aids, and early recognition of dehydration were components of the intervention group. Another randomized study compared postoperative usual care with care given in a specialized geriatric ward after hip fracture surgery. The interventions were numerous, but included an almost 1:1 nurse/aide-to-patient ratio, staff education, interdisciplinary teams, individual care planning, active prevention of complications, including urinary tract infections, constipation, falls, anemia, supplemental oxygen, active nutrition, and early mobilization. The intervention group experienced an absolute risk reduction of 20.4%; the duration of delirium was almost half that of controls, and they remained in the hospital for fewer number of days.[6] Combining pre- and postoperative geriatric assessments, early surgery, supplemental oxygen, close monitoring of blood pressure to reduce hypotension, and treatment of postoperative complications for hip fracture patients reduced the incidence, severity, and duration of delirium episodes, but this study was not randomized.[89]

Geriatric consultation alone reduces the incidence of delirium. A randomized trial of hip fracture patients comparing proactive geriatric consultation with usual care resulted in a number needed to treat of 5.6 patients to prevent 1 case of delirium, and the reduction was more robust in preventing severe delirium.[90] On average, 9.5 recommendations were made for each patient, relating to oxygen delivery, environmental modifications, fluid/electrolyte management, pain, medications, bowel/bladder function, nutrition, mobilization, prevention, detection and treatment of complications, and treatment of agitation. Other studies corroborate the benefits of a perioperative comprehensive geriatric assessment.[91]

Environmental modifications may influence delirium rates. Interventions as simple as music therapy during the postoperative period reduce the rates of delirium.[92] One study reported higher incidence of delirium in the winter,[93] suggesting that access to sunlight may be important. Improving ward conditions with spacious rooms, community dining, and unrestricted visiting hours, and encouraging family members to visit and bring familiar items from home are beneficial.[94]

Improving staff awareness, education, and continuity is valuable. Although no reduction in the incidence of delirium was seen, educating the nursing staff, systematically screening all patients, and using a pain-management protocol decreased the duration of delirium episodes in 1 nonrandomized trial.[95] Improving continuity of care has been implemented as part of multifactorial strategies,[94] but the data on the benefit of this intervention are limited.

Several methods to restore normal sleep–wake cycles have been studied. Bright light therapy had no effect on the incidence of delirium in 1 small, randomized study.[96] In another prospective, randomized trial, administration of flunitrazepam, pethidine (meperidine), and diazepam postoperatively resulted in an absolute risk reduction of 30% for developing delirium.[97] However, these medications can precipitate delirium and generally are not recommended for use in the elderly.[33,36,42,50,78,82,98] Lastly, case reports suggest that melatonin might be helpful in the prevention and treatment of delirium.[99]

Various medications have been prescribed in an attempt to reduce the incidence of delirium. A randomized trial of patients who underwent elective cardiac surgery demonstrated an absolute risk reduction of 20.6% when the patients were given 1 mg of risperidone once on awakening.[100] Haloperidol, 1.5 mg daily, did not reduce the incidence of delirium, but the severity and duration of symptoms were decreased.[101] As an adjunctive pain medication and opioid-sparing agent, gabapentin, 900 mg daily, significantly reduced the incidence of postoperative delirium, but this study enrolled only 21 patients with a mean age of about 60 years.[102] Two small studies randomized participants to donepezil 5 mg daily or placebo before elective orthopedic surgery and found no difference in the rates of postoperative delirium.[103,104]

In addition to the immediate benefits, preventive strategies reduce subsequent health care costs. Leslie and colleagues[105] followed patients, who had participated in a randomized study aimed at the prevention of delirium, for 1 year. Although both intervention and control arms had similar rates of long-term institutionalization, those in the intervention group used 15.7% fewer health care dollars (almost $10,000 less annually), primarily because of shorter duration of nursing home stays (mean stay: 241 days for intervention group vs. 280 days for usual care).

CLINICAL PRESENTATION

Hallmarks of delirium include inattention, disorientation, and disorganized thinking. Patients may be aware of their delirium and report confusion. The onset is acute, and impairments fluctuate within the course of a day. Altered behavior, memory problems, irritability, changes in sleep cycle, and hallucinations may also occur.

Three categories of delirium exist: hyperactive, hypoactive, and mixed.[106] Psychomotor agitation characterizes the hyperactive form, which can be accompanied by diaphoresis, tachycardia, xerostomia, mydriasis, tremor, and combativeness. These manifestations are more commonly identified early in the course, as they often disrupt and interfere with medical care. The hypoactive form, less easily recognized,[107] consists of low psychomotor activity and somnolence. Hallucinations, perceptual disturbances, and delusions occur with either subtype.[108] A systematic review of 10 studies revealed no consensus as to which type is more common in medical and surgical geriatric patients.[109] Some studies report that after hip surgery hypoactive delirium is more common,[110] whereas others report a higher proportion of the hyperactive form.[111] This discrepancy may be because of the lack of a standardized assessment tool to differentiate among the subtypes of delirium.[109]

DIAGNOSIS

The American Psychiatric Association describes the diagnostic criteria for delirium in the *Diagnostic and Statistical Manual of Mental Disorders, Fourth Edition, Text Revision* (DSM-IV-TR).[112] The diagnostic criteria for delirium include the following: (1) disturbance of consciousness (ie, reduced clarity of awareness of the environment) with reduced ability to focus, sustain, or shift attention; (2) a change in cognition (such as memory deficit, disorientation, and language disturbance) or the development of a perceptual disturbance that is not better accounted for by a preexisting, established, or evolving dementia; (3) development of the disturbance over a short period of time (usually hours to days), with a tendency for it to fluctuate during the course of the day; and (4) there is evidence from the history, physical examination, or laboratory findings that the disturbance is caused by the direct physiological consequences of a general medical condition.

Delirium is a clinical diagnosis without a "gold standard" diagnostic test. Initial laboratory investigation should include a complete blood count, electrolytes, blood urea nitrogen, creatinine, glucose, calcium, magnesium, phosphorus, hepatic function panel, urinalysis, arterial blood gas, ECG, and chest radiograph.[113] Abnormalities on the ECG should prompt analysis of serial cardiac enzymes, even in the absence of cardiac symptoms, such as chest pain or shortness of breath. Findings on history and physical examination should guide further laboratory investigation, such as urine toxicology screen or serum levels of medications. An electroencephalogram may be useful if seizure disorder is suspected.[30] Neuroimaging is indicated when focal neurologic deficits are identified or there is a history of head trauma.[30] Given that postoperative stroke incidence increases with age[114,115] and acute stroke is often associated with delirium,[116] neuroimaging may be useful in evaluating for a new stroke or intracranial hemorrhage even in the absence of new neurologic deficits.

Various delirium-screening instruments exist for clinical and research use (**Table 2**). A comparison of 13 instruments recommends the NEECHAM confusion scale (NCS, named after its developers Neelon and Champagne) and delirium observation screening (DOS) scale for screening high-risk, hospitalized elderly patients.[117] The NCS is the only instrument to include physiologic parameters, such as vital sign stability and urinary incontinence, and the scale is 86% to 100% sensitive and 86% to 90% specific.[118,119] The DOS is easy to use and, therefore, is preferred over the NCS; the DOS is 89% sensitive and 88% specific.[119,120]

The Confusion Assessment Method (CAM), considered the best diagnostic tool,[117] looks for the following features: (1) inattention, (2) acute onset and fluctuating course, (3) altered level of consciousness, and (4) disorganized thinking. When patients show features 1 and 2 and either feature 3 or 4, the CAM is 94% to 100% sensitive and 90% to 95% specific for diagnosing delirium.[121] All the aforementioned instruments require a verbal patient; hence, the CAM-ICU was developed for ventilated patients; it has 93% to 100% sensitivity and 98% to 100% specificity compared with expert diagnosis of delirium.[122]

The Delirium Rating Scale-revised-98 (DRS-R-98) is yet another tool that is 91% to 100% sensitive and 85% to 100% specific in diagnosing delirium and distinguishing it from dementia, depression, and schizophrenia.[123] Observations of sleep–wake cycle, perceptual disturbances and hallucinations, delusions, lability of affect, language, thought processes, motor agitation or retardation, orientation, attention, short- and long-term memory, visuospatial ability, temporal onset of symptoms, fluctuations in symptom severity, and underlying physiologic, medical, or pharmacologic disorders are included. Although more time-consuming than the CAM, the added benefit of the DRS-R-98 is that it evaluates delirium severity and is helpful in the context of prior psychiatric disorders.[123]

Despite sensitive and specific screening tests, delirium remains underrecognized[107] with up to two thirds of cases being missed by physicians.[30] One study revealed that requests for psychiatric consultation for depression were actually delirium or dementia in up to 52% of referrals.[124] Inouye and colleagues[107] demonstrated that nurses were more likely to miss the diagnosis of delirium if patients exhibited the hypoactive form, had dementia, had vision impairment, or were 80 years or older. Many of these variables are characteristics that place patients at a higher risk for developing delirium. Inouye and colleagues[107] estimated that patients with 3 or 4 risk factors for delirium have a 20-fold risk for delirium underrecognition by nurses. Staff training may be another factor; 1 study suggests that the sensitivity of the CAM depends on the training background of the operator.[125]

MANAGEMENT

Identification and treatment of the underlying causes of delirium are essential. This remains a difficult task, given that there may be many contributing factors, and the elderly often present with nonspecific findings. In one study of delirium after hip fracture surgery, only 7% were assigned a definite cause and 61% were presumed to be related to a comorbid condition. In addition, 74 identifiable causes were attributable to the 33 comorbid cases, suggesting that, frequently, there is more than one causative factor.[126] A careful review of the patient's medication list is of paramount importance.[30] Apart from treating the underlying condition, management strategies are categorized into supportive measures and symptom control.

Supportive measures are geared toward maintaining patient safety and include many of the preventive strategies. A multidisciplinary approach emphasizing frequent reorientation, appropriate

Table 2
Comparison of common screening and diagnostic instruments

Instrument	Variables Evaluated	Comments
Neecham Confusion Scale (NCS)[118,119]	• Processing—attention, following commands, orientation • Behavior—appearance, motor, verbal • Physiology—vital signs, urinary continence • Systolic BP <100 or >160 • Diastolic BP <50 or >90 • Heart rate <60 or >100 bpm • Respiratory rate <14 or >22 per min • Room air oxygen saturation <93%	• Only instrument to include physiologic parameters • 86%–100% sensitive • 86%–90% specific
Delirium Observation Screening Scale (DOS)[119,120]	• Intermittent somnolence • Easily distracted • Attention • Gives incomplete answers • Gives inappropriate answers • Reaction time • Oriented to place • Oriented to time • Short-term memory • Restlessness • Agitation • Labile affect • Perceptual disturbances	• Initial scale included 25 items, which was modified to 13 items • Takes <5 min to complete • 89% sensitive • 88% specific
Confusion Assessment Method (CAM)[121]	• Inattention • Acute onset and fluctuating course and • Altered level of consciousness or • Disorganized thinking	• Most commonly used • Takes <5 min to complete • 94%–100% sensitive • 90%–95% specific
Delirium Rating Scale-Revised-98 (DRS-R-98)[123]	• Sleep–wake cycle disturbance • Perceptual disturbances and hallucinations • Delusions • Lability of affect • Language • Thought-process abnormalities • Motor agitation • Motor retardation • Orientation • Attention • Short-term memory • Long-term memory • Visuospatial ability • Temporal onset of symptoms • Fluctuations in symptom severity • Physical disorder	• Also assesses severity of symptoms • 91%–100% sensitive • 85%–100% specific

Abbreviations: BP, blood pressure; bpm, beats per minute.

stimulation, environmental safety, and patient comfort is crucial. Geriatric consultation may help modify known risk factors. Physical restraints should be avoided because they may worsen confusion; use of restraints placed patients at a fourfold higher risk for developing delirium in 1 study.[31] A one-on-one companion is often helpful in reorienting the patient and ensuring safety.

Symptom control for agitation and aggression may be necessary to ensure patient and staff safety, but such measures should not delay the diagnosis of an underlying cause. Antipsychotics are first-line, with haloperidol being the preferred agent because of its minimal anticholinergic side effects and lack of active metabolites. Starting doses of as low as 0.25 to 0.50 mg every 4 hours as needed are recommended in the elderly.[113] Only a few trials have compared haloperidol with the newer, atypical antipsychotics, and a meta-analysis revealed no difference in efficacy and tolerability between low-dose haloperidol and olanzapine or risperidone.[127]

Benzodiazepines are not recommended to treat delirium unless the underlying cause is withdrawal from alcohol or benzodiazepines.[113] Lorazepam, with its short half-life and absence of active metabolites, is preferred in the elderly, with starting doses of as low as 0.5 mg. If both antipsychotics and benzodiazepines are used, the doses of each should be decreased because they work synergistically.

Given the side-effect profiles of antipsychotics and benzodiazepines, studies have been conducted on other medications to treat delirium. Intravenous administration of the serotonin receptor antagonist ondansetron to postoperative delirious patients resulted in improvements in consciousness, awareness, and agitation.[128] However, this was a nonrandomized, nonblinded study, the delirium diagnostic tool was not validated, and long-lasting improvements in mental status were not evaluated. Case reports suggest that cholinergics, such as physostigmine, may be useful in delirium known to be caused specifically by anticholinergic medications.[129]

Lastly, patient and family education on delirium should take place.[113] The experience takes a psychological toll on patients and families, especially when psychotic symptoms occur. Emphasizing the temporary nature of the condition, its reversibility, and its relationship to the underlying cause are critically important. Limited data exist on the effectiveness of these efforts, but surveys of family members of patients with terminal delirium in palliative care units suggest they are helpful.[130]

OUTCOMES

Mortality is higher for those who experience postoperative delirium,[2,3] in the immediate postoperative setting[7] and up to 1 year after surgery.[4] Morbidity in the medical, functional, psychological, and social domains is also affected.

Patients with postoperative delirium are at increased risk for experiencing other medical postoperative complications.[2,5] Studies show higher rates of falls, pressure ulcers, urinary infections, wound infections, aspiration, pneumonia, need for urinary catheters, malnutrition, perioperative myocardial infarction, and atrial fibrillation.[6–8] Delirious patients often require longer intubations and re-intubations,[7,10] use more hospital resources, spend longer time in the intensive care unit,[5,9,10] and remain in the hospital longer than their nondelirious counterparts.[3,5,10,13,42,59]

Postoperative delirium increases the risk for subsequent functional loss and institutionalization. Fewer delirious patients are able to continue living at home[11] or with family members[5] after hospital discharge, and many require nursing home placement,[2] confirming the association between delirium and loss of independence. Six months after hip fracture surgery, those with delirium are more likely to have reduced walking ability[2,8] and be wheelchair-bound or bedridden.[11] Delirious patients experience subsequent decline in ADLs,[2] which persists even a year after surgery.[4]

Postoperative delirium is a risk factor for subsequent cognitive decline. Confusion can remain for up to 6 months after an episode of delirium.[2] Delirious patients are more likely to experience a decline in subsequent MMSE scores[12] and have a higher likelihood of developing dementia.[13] It is possible that some patients have unrecognized preexisting cognitive impairment, which the delirium unmasks, but most studies report preoperative MMSE scores indicating normal cognitive function.

Quality-of-life measures are affected during and after an episode of delirium. Patients with delirium are more likely to report sleep dissatisfaction[14] and insomnia[8] in the immediate postoperative period.[14] They are at risk for more episodes of subsequent delirium and are more likely to be depressed.[8] Lower self-rated well-being[8] and declines in health-related quality of life[12] persist for up to 6 months after delirium. Lastly, a study of delirious cancer patients found that most patients recall their delirious episodes, and when they do, they suffer subsequent psychological distress as do their family members and caregivers.[15]

RECOMMENDATIONS AND CONCLUSIONS

Modeling of the preventive multidisciplinary strategies used in trials is ideal but not always feasible. Interventions that can be implemented by a surgical team preoperatively and postoperatively are listed in **Box 1**. In addition, specific diagnostic

Box 1
Summary of recommended perioperative actions for the surgical team

Preoperative actions

- Assess baseline risk with MMSE or clock drawing test
- Optimize vital signs (BP, oxygen saturation)
- Treat electrolyte imbalances
- Maintain glycemic control
- Monitor volume status
- Geriatric consultation for vulnerable elderly undergoing major surgery
- Consider psychiatric consultation for evaluation and treatment of depression

Postoperative actions

- Optimize awareness of and interaction with environment
- Ensure adequate pain control
- Avoid meperidine, benzodiazepines, and anticholinergics (diphenhydramine)
- Ensure early ambulation
- Remove urinary catheters as soon as possible

tools and treatment plans based on a review of the literature are presented in **Box 2**.

In the preoperative period, recognition of predisposing factors, although usually nonmodifiable, is essential to identify patients at risk for developing postoperative delirium. A Folstein MMSE or clock-drawing test should become part of the routine preoperative assessment to assess cognitive impairment. Additionally, vital signs, such as blood pressure and oxygen saturation before surgery should be stabilized, electrolyte imbalances (especially disorders of sodium and potassium) should be identified and treated, reasonable glycemic control should be enforced, and volume status should be monitored. Geriatric consultation should be requested for vulnerable elderly patients undergoing major surgery, especially orthopedic and cardiac procedures. Vulnerability includes poor self-rated health, functional disabilities (such as ADL impairment), limitations in physical functioning (such as difficulty carrying 10 lb or walking one-quarter of a mile), and age older than 75 years.[131] For these patients, preoperative geriatric consultation can assist in identifying the risk factors for postsurgical complications and suggest preventive strategies. In addition, recommendations based on the Assessing Care of Vulnerable Elders Project Quality Indicators[132] specific to medication management, pain control, bowel and bladder function, nutrition, and mobilization may benefit patients. Lastly, the team should consider psychiatric consultation for evaluation and treatment of depression, although this may be more helpful in the weeks before surgery rather than in the days preceding the operation.

In the postoperative period, the patient's awareness of and interaction with his or her environment should be optimized through the use of visual aids, hearing aids, familiar visitors, frequent reorientation, and access to sunlight. Ensuring adequate pain control is essential; the use of opioids may be necessary, but meperidine should be avoided. Other medications, such as benzodiazepines and anticholinergics, especially diphenhydramine, are equally dangerous for the elderly patient. Ambulation should occur as soon as possible, along with prompt removal of urinary catheters.

Timely diagnosis of delirium necessitates a high index of suspicion on the part of the surgical team. Any change in clinical or mental status should prompt a thorough investigation. Of the many diagnostic instruments available, the authors recommend the CAM. Searching for the underlying causes is a necessary component of the diagnostic endeavor.

Regarding management strategies, the priorities are ensuring appropriate nutrition and hydration and emphasizing patient safety while treating the underlying causes. Restraints should be avoided and a one-on-one companion should be considered instead. When medications are required for agitation or aggression, low doses of haloperidol (0.25–0.5 mg) should be given and titrated to symptom control. The patient and his or her family should be educated about the condition and its expected course.

Box 2
Diagnostic and treatment recommendations for the surgical team

Diagnosis

- Maintain high index of suspicion
- Use the CAM for quick and accurate diagnosis
- Investigate for underlying causes

Treatment strategies

- Treat the underlying causes
- Emphasize patient safety
- Ensure adequate nutrition and hydration
- Avoid restraints; consider ordering one-on-one companion
- Use low-dose haloperidol for symptom control
- Educate patient and family

In summary, postoperative delirium commonly afflicts the geriatric population, but is often unrecognized despite sensitive and specific screening and diagnostic instruments. Predisposing and precipitating factors interact to confer risk for developing postoperative delirium, and it is both helpful and feasible for the surgical team to implement preventive strategies aimed at modifying those risk factors. Management consists of treating the underlying causes, providing supportive measures, and using antipsychotics for agitation. The consequences of postoperative delirium can be devastating and impact mortality and morbidity in the medical, functional, psychological, and socioeconomic domains. Improving recognition and treatment of this condition will benefit patients and mitigate a significant economic burden.

ACKNOWLEDGMENTS

The authors thank Bernard Roos, MD, for thoughtful critique and Virginia Roos for assistance in editing the manuscript.

REFERENCES

1. Brown TM, Boyle MF. Delirium. BMJ 2002;325(7365):644–7.
2. Marcantonio ER, Flacker JM, Michaels M, et al. Delirium is independently associated with poor functional recovery after hip fracture. J Am Geriatr Soc 2000;48(6):618–24.
3. Rudolph JL, Jones RN, Rasmussen LS, et al. Independent vascular and cognitive risk factors for postoperative delirium. Am J Med 2007;120(9):807–13.
4. Edelstein DM, Aharonoff GB, Karp A, et al. Effect of postoperative delirium on outcome after hip fracture. Clin Orthop Relat Res 2004;422:195–200.
5. Zakriya K, Sieber FE, Christmas C, et al. Brief postoperative delirium in hip fracture patients affects functional outcome at three months. Anesth Analg 2004;98(6):1798–802.
6. Lundstrom M, Olofsson B, Stenvall M, et al. Postoperative delirium in old patients with femoral neck fracture: a randomized intervention study. Aging Clin Exp Res 2007;19(3):178–86.
7. Norkiene I, Ringaitiene D, Misiuriene I, et al. Incidence and precipitating factors of delirium after coronary artery bypass grafting. Scand Cardiovasc J 2007;41(3):180–5.
8. Olofsson B, Lundström M, Borssén B, et al. Delirium is associated with poor rehabilitation outcome in elderly patients treated for femoral neck fractures. Scand J Caring Sci 2005;19(2):119–27.
9. Böhner H, Hummel TC, Habel U, et al. Predicting delirium after vascular surgery. A model based on pre- and intraoperative data. Ann Surg 2003;238(1):149–56.
10. Bucerius J, Gummert JF, Borger MA, et al. Predictors of delirium after cardiac surgery delirium: effect of beating-heart (off-pump) surgery. J Thorac Cardiovasc Surg 2004;127(1):57–64.
11. Edlund A, Lundström M, Lundström G, et al. Clinical profile of delirium in patients treated for femoral neck fractures. Dement Geriatr Cogn Disord 1999;10(5):325–9.
12. Duppils GS, Wikblad K. Cognitive function and health-related quality of life after delirium in connection with hip surgery. A six-month follow-up. Orthop Nurs 2004;23(3):195–203.
13. Lundström M, Edlund A, Bucht G, et al. Dementia after delirium in patients with femoral neck fractures. J Am Geriatr Soc 2003;51(7):1002–6.
14. Bowman AM. Sleep satisfaction, perceived pain and acute confusion in elderly clients undergoing orthopaedic procedures. J Adv Nurs 1997;26(3):550–64.
15. Breitbart W, Gibson C, Tremblay A. The delirium experience: delirium recall and delirium-related distress in hospitalized patients with cancer, their spouses/caregivers, and their nurses. Psychosomatics 2002;43(3):183–94.
16. Department of Health and Human Services. 2004 CMS Statistics. CMS publication no. 03445. Washington, DC: Department of Health and Human Services; 2004.
17. Leslie DL, Marcantonio ER, Zhang Y, et al. One-year health care costs associated with delirium in the elderly population. Arch Intern Med 2008;168(1):27–32.
18. Mussi C, Ferrari R, Ascari S, et al. Importance of serum anticholinergic activity in the assessment of elderly patients with delirium. J Geriatr Psychiatry Neurol 1999;12(2):82–6.
19. Uchida K, Aoki T, Ishizuka B. Postoperative delirium and plasma melatonin. Med Hypotheses 1999;53(2):103–6.
20. Balan S, Leibovitz A, Zila SO, et al. The relation between the clinical subtypes of delirium and the urinary level of 6-SMT. J Neuropsychiatry Clin Neurosci 2003;15(3):363–6.
21. Lewis MC, Barnett SR. Postoperative delirium: the tryptophan dysregulation model. Med Hypotheses 2004;63(3):402–6.
22. Nakamura J, Yoshimura R, Okuno T, et al. Association of plasma free-3-methoxy-4-hydroxyphenyl (ethylene)glycol, natural killer cell activity and delirium in postoperative patients. Int Clin Psychopharmacol 2001;16(6):339–43.
23. Karlidag R, Unal S, Sezer OH, et al. The role of oxidative stress in postoperative delirium. Gen Hosp Psychiatry 2006;28(5):418–23.

24. Rudolph JL, Ramlawi B, Kuchel GA, et al. Chemokines are associated with delirium after cardiac surgery. J Gerontol A Biol Sci Med Sci 2008; 63A(2):184–9.
25. de Rooij SE, van Munster BC, Korevaar JC, et al. Cytokines and acute phase response in delirium. J Psychosom Res 2007;62(5):521–5.
26. Hala M. Pathophysiology of postoperative delirium: systemic inflammation as a response to surgical trauma causes diffuse microcirculatory impairment. Med Hypotheses 2007;68(1):194–6.
27. Plaschke K, Hill H, Engelhardt R, et al. EEG changes and serum anticholinergic activity measured in patients with delirium in the intensive care unit. Anaesthesia 2007;62(12):1217–23.
28. Yokota H, Ogawa S, Kurokawa A, et al. Regional cerebral blood flow in delirium patients. Psychiatry Clin Neurosci 2003;57(3):337–9.
29. Inouye SK. Predisposing and precipitating factors for delirium in hospitalized older patients. Dement Geriatr Cogn Disord 1999;10(5):393–400.
30. Inouye SK, Charpentier PA. Precipitating factors for delirium in hospitalized elderly persons. Predictive model and interrelationship with baseline vulnerability. J Am Med Assoc 1996;275(11):852–7.
31. Inouye SK. The dilemma of delirium: clinical and research controversies regarding diagnosis and evaluation of delirium in hospitalized elderly medical patients. Am J Med 1994;97(3):278–88.
32. Eriksson M, Samuelsson E, Gustafson Y, et al. Delirium after coronary bypass surgery evaluated by the organic brain syndrome protocol. Scand Cardiovasc J 2002;36(4):250–5.
33. Leung JM, Sands LP, Vaurio LE, et al. Nitrous oxide does not change the incidence of postoperative delirium or cognitive decline in elderly surgical patients. Br J Anaesth 2006;96(6):754–60.
34. Williams-Russo P, Urquhart BL, Sharrock NE, et al. Post-operative delirium: predictors and prognosis in elderly orthopedic patients. J Am Geriatr Soc 1992;40(8):759–67.
35. Lynch EP, Lazor MA, Gellis JE, et al. The impact of postoperative pain on the development of postoperative delirium. Anesth Analg 1998;86(4): 781–5.
36. Morrison RS, Magaziner J, Gilbert M, et al. Relationship between pain and opioid analgesics on the development of delirium following hip fracture. J Gerontol A Biol Sci Med Sci 2003;58A(1):76–81.
37. Marcantonio ER, Goldman L, Mangione CM, et al. A clinical prediction rule for delirium after elective noncardiac surgery. J Am Med Assoc 1994; 271(2):134–9.
38. Galanakis P, Bickel H, Gradinger R, et al. Acute confusional state in the elderly following hip surgery: incidence, risk factors and complications. Int J Geriatr Psychiatry 2001;16(4):349–55.
39. Sasajima Y, Sasajima T, Uchida H, et al. Postoperative delirium in patients with chronic lower limb ischaemia: what are the specific markers? Eur J Vasc Endovasc Surg 2000;20(2):132–7.
40. Yıldızeli B, Özyurtkan MO, Batırel HF, et al. Factors associated with postoperative delirium after thoracic surgery. Ann Thorac Surg 2005;79(3):1004–9.
41. Kalisvaart KJ, Vreeswijk R, de Jonghe JF, et al. Risk factors and prediction of postoperative delirium in elderly hip-surgery patients: implementation and validation of a medical risk factor model. J Am Geriatr Soc 2006;54(5):817–22.
42. Litaker D, Locala J, Franco K, et al. Preoperative risk factors for postoperative delirium. Gen Hosp Psychiatry 2001;23(2):84–9.
43. Vaurio LE, Sands LP, Wang Y, et al. Postoperative delirium: the importance of pain and pain management. Anesth Analg 2006;102(4):1267–73.
44. Resnick N. Geriatric medicine. In: Braunwald E, Fauci A, Kasper D, et al, editors. Harrison's principles of internal medicine. 15th edition. New York: McGraw-Hill; 2001. p. 36–46.
45. Tagarakis GI, Tsolaki-Tagaraki F, Tsolaki M, et al. The role of apolipoprotein E in cognitive decline and delirium after bypass heart operations. Am J Alzheimers Dis Other Demen 2007;22(3):223–8.
46. Endo Y, Aharonoff GB, Zuckerman JD, et al. Gender differences in patients with hip fracture: a greater risk of morbidity and mortality in men. J Orthop Trauma 2005;19(1):29–35.
47. Fisher BW, Flowerdew G. A simple model for predicting postoperative delirium in older patients undergoing elective orthopedic surgery. J Am Geriatr Soc 1995;43(2):175–8.
48. Papaioannou A, Fraidakis O, Michaloudis D, et al. The impact of the type of anaesthesia on cognitive status and delirium during the first postoperative days in elderly patients. Eur J Anaesthesiol 2005; 22(7):492–9.
49. Zakriya KJ, Christmas C, Wenz JF Sr, et al. Preoperative factors associated with postoperative change in confusion assessment method score in hip fracture patients. Anesth Analg 2002;94(6): 1628–32.
50. Benoit AG, Campbell BI, Tanner JR, et al. Risk factors and prevalence of perioperative cognitive dysfunction in abdominal aneurysm patients. J Vasc Surg 2005;42(5):884–90.
51. Fukuse T, Satoda N, Hijiya K, et al. Importance of a comprehensive geriatric assessment in prediction of complications following thoracic surgery in elderly patients. Chest 2005;127(3):886–91.
52. Veliz-Reissmüller G, Agüero Torres H, van der Linden J, et al. Pre-operative mild cognitive dysfunction predicts risk for post-operative delirium after elective cardiac surgery. Aging Clin Exp Res 2007;19(3):172–7.

53. Fick DM, Agostini JV, Inouye SK. Delirium superimposed on dementia: a systematic review. J Am Geriatr Soc 2002;50(10):1723–32.
54. Rudolph JL, Jones RN, Grande LJ, et al. Impaired executive function is associated with delirium after coronary artery bypass graft surgery. J Am Geriatr Soc 2006;54(6):937–41.
55. Lowery DP, Wesnes K, Ballard CG. Subtle attentional deficits in the absence of dementia are associated with an increased risk of post-operative delirium. Dement Geriatr Cogn Disord 2007;23(6):390–4.
56. Jones RN, Yang FM, Zhang Y, et al. Does educational attainment contribute to risk for delirium? A potential role for cognitive reserve. J Gerontol A Biol Sci Med Sci 2006;61A(12):1307–11.
57. Rudolph JL, Babikian VL, Birjiniuk V, et al. Atherosclerosis is associated with delirium after coronary artery bypass graft surgery. J Am Geriatr Soc 2005;53(3):462–6.
58. Olofsson B, Stenvall M, Lundström M, et al. Malnutrition in hip fracture patients: an intervention study. J Clin Nurs 2007;16(11):2027–38.
59. Berggren D, Gustafson Y, Eriksson B, et al. Postoperative confusion after anesthesia in elderly patients with femoral neck fractures. Anesth Analg 1987;66(6):497–504.
60. Leung JM, Sands LP, Mullen EA, et al. Are preoperative depressive symptoms associated with postoperative delirium in geriatric surgical patients? J Gerontol A Biol Sci Med Sci 2005;60A(12):1563–8.
61. Simpson CJ, Kellett JM. The relationship between pre-operative anxiety and post-operative delirium. J Psychosom Res 1987;31(4):491–7.
62. Aakerlund LP, Rosenberg J. Postoperative delirium: treatment with supplementary oxygen. Br J Anaesth 1994;72(3):286–90.
63. Leung JM, Sands LP, Wang Y, et al. Apolipoprotein E e4 allele increases the risk of early postoperative delirium in older patients undergoing noncardiac surgery. Anesthesiology 2007;107(3):406–11.
64. Bitsch MS, Foss NB, Kristensen BB, et al. Pathogenesis of and management strategies for postoperative delirium after hip fracture. A review. Acta Orthop Scand 2004;75(4):378–89.
65. Balasundaram B, Holmes J. Delirium in vascular surgery. Eur J Vasc Endovasc Surg 2007;34(2):131–4.
66. Seymour DG, Vaz FG. A prospective study of elderly general surgical patients: II. Post-operative complications. Age Ageing 1989;18(5):316–26.
67. Mann C, Pouzeratte Y, Boccara G, et al. Comparison of intravenous or epidural patient-controlled analgesia in the elderly after major abdominal surgery. Anesthesiology 2000;92(2):433–41.
68. Milstein A, Pollack A, Kleinman G, et al. Confusion/delirium following cataract surgery: an incidence study of 1-year duration. Int Psychogeriatr 2002;14(3):301–6.
69. Chaudhuri S, Mahar RS, Gurunadh VS. Delirium after cataract extraction: a prospective study. J Indian Med Assoc 1994;92(8):268–9.
70. Bruce AJ, Ritchie CW, Blizard R, et al. The incidence of delirium associated with orthopedic surgery: a meta-analytic review. Int Psychogeriatr 2007;19(2):197–214.
71. Agnoletti V, Ansaloni L, Catena F, et al. Postoperative delirium after elective and emergency surgery: analysis and checking of risk factors. A study protocol. BMC Surg 2005;5:1–6.
72. Marcantonio ER, Goldman L, Orav EJ, et al. The association of intraoperative factors with the development of postoperative delirium. Am J Med 1998;105(5):380–4.
73. Nishikawa K, Nakayama M, Omote K, et al. Recovery characteristics and post-operative delirium after long-duration laparoscope-assisted surgery in elderly patients: propofol-based vs. sevoflurane-based anesthesia. Acta Anaesthesiol Scand 2004;48(2):162–8.
74. Inouye SK. Prevention of delirium in hospitalized older patients: risk factors and targeted intervention strategies. Annu Mediaev 2000;32(4):257–63.
75. Kamel HK, Iqbal MA, Mogallapu R, et al. Time to ambulation after hip fracture surgery: relation to hospitalization outcomes. J Gerontol A Biol Sci Med Sci 2003;58A(11):1042–5.
76. Beaussier M, Weickmans H, Parc Y, et al. Postoperative analgesia and recovery course after major colorectal surgery in elderly patients: a randomized comparison between intrathecal morphine and intravenous PCA morphine. Reg Anesth Pain Med 2006;31(6):531–8.
77. Chilvers CR, Nguyen MH, Robertson IK. Changing from epidural to multimodal analgesia for colorectal laparotomy: an audit. Anaesth Intensive Care 2007;35(2):230–8.
78. Marcantonio ER, Juarez G, Goldman L, et al. The relationship of postoperative delirium with psychoactive medications. J Am Med Assoc 1994;272(19):1518–22.
79. Tune LE. Serum anticholinergic activity levels and delirium in the elderly. Semin Clin Neuropsychiatry 2000;5(2):149–53.
80. Han L, McCusker J, Cole M, et al. Use of medications with anticholinergic effect predicts clinical severity of delirium symptoms in older medical inpatients. Arch Intern Med 2001;161(8):1099–105.
81. Agostini JV, Leo-Summers LS, Inouye SK. Cognitive and other adverse effects of diphenhydramine use in hospitalized older patients. Arch Intern Med 2001;161(17):2091–7.

82. Adunsky A, Levy R, Heim M, et al. Meperidine analgesia and delirium in aged hip fracture patients. Arch Gerontol Geriatr 2002;35(3):253–9.
83. Fong HK, Sands LP, Leung JM. The role of postoperative analgesia in delirium and cognitive decline in elderly patients: a systematic review. Anesth Analg 2006;102(4):1255–66.
84. Herrick IA, Ganapathy S, Komar W, et al. Postoperative cognitive impairment in the elderly. Choice of patient-controlled analgesia opioid. Anaesthesia 1996;51(4):356–60.
85. Rapp SE, Egan KJ, Ross BK, et al. A multidimensional comparison of morphine and hydromorphone patient-controlled analgesia. Anesth Analg 1996;82(5):1043–8.
86. Silvasti M, Svartling N, Pitkänen M, et al. Comparison of intravenous patient-controlled analgesia with tramadol versus morphine after microvascular breast reconstruction. Eur J Anaesthesiol 2000; 17(7):448–55.
87. Inouye SK, Schlesinger MJ, Lydon TJ. Delirium: a symptom of how hospital care is failing older persons and a window to improve quality of hospital care. Am J Med 1999;106(5):565–73.
88. Inouye SK, Bogardus ST Jr, Charpentier PA, et al. A multicomponent intervention to prevent delirium in hospitalized older patients. N Engl J Med 1999; 340(9):669–76.
89. Gustafson Y, Brännström B, Berggren D, et al. A geriatric-anesthesiologic program to reduce acute confusional states in elderly patients treated for femoral neck fractures. J Am Geriatr Soc 1991; 39(7):655–62.
90. Marcantonio ER, Flacker JM, Wright RJ, et al. Reducing delirium after hip fracture: a randomized trial. J Am Geriatr Soc 2001;49(5):516–22.
91. Harari D, Hopper A, Dhesi J, et al. Proactive care of older people undergoing surgery ('POPS'): designing, embedding, evaluating and funding a comprehensive geriatric assessment service for older elective surgical patients. Age Ageing 2007; 36(2):190–6.
92. Ruth M, Locsin R. The effect of music listening on acute confusion and delirium in elders undergoing elective hip and knee surgery. J Clin Nurs 2004; 13(6b):91–6.
93. Balan S, Leibovitz A, Freedman L, et al. Seasonal variation in the incidence of delirium among the patients of a geriatric hospital. Arch Gerontol Geriatr 2001;33(3):287–93.
94. Lundström M, Edlund A, Lundström G, et al. Reorganization of nursing and medical care to reduce the incidence of postoperative delirium and improve rehabilitation outcome in elderly patients treated for femoral neck fractures. Scand J Caring Sci 1998;13(3):193–200.
95. Milisen K, Foreman MD, Abraham IL, et al. A nurse-led interdisciplinary intervention program for delirium in elderly hip-fracture patients. J Am Geriatr Soc 2001;49(5):523–32.
96. Taguchi T, Yano M, Kido Y. Influence of bright light therapy on postoperative patients: a pilot study. Intensive Crit Care Nurs 2007;23(5):289–97.
97. Aizawa K, Kanai T, Saikawa Y, et al. A novel approach to the prevention of postoperative delirium in the elderly after gastrointestinal surgery. Surg Today 2002;32(4):310–4.
98. Beers MH. Explicit criteria for determining potentially inappropriate medication use by the elderly. An update. Arch Intern Med 1997;157(14):1531–6.
99. Hanania M, Kitain E. Melatonin for treatment and prevention of postoperative delirium. Anesth Analg 2002;94(2):338–9.
100. Prakanrattana U, Prapaitrakool S. Efficacy of risperidone for prevention of postoperative delirium in cardiac surgery. Anaesth Intensive Care 2007; 35(5):714–9.
101. Kalisvaart KJ, de Jonghe JF, Bogaards MJ, et al. Haloperidol prophylaxis for elderly hip-surgery patients at risk for delirium: a randomized placebo-controlled study. J Am Geriatr Soc 2005; 53(10):1658–66.
102. Leung JM, Sands LP, Rico M, et al. Pilot clinical trial of gabapentin to decrease postoperative delirium in older patients. Neurology 2006;67(7):1251–3.
103. Liptzin B, Laki A, Garb JL, et al. Donepezil in the prevention and treatment of post-surgical delirium. Am J Geriatr Psychiatry 2005;13(12):1100–6.
104. Sampson EL, Raven PR, Ndhlovu PN, et al. A randomized, double-blind, placebo-controlled trial of donepezil hydrochloride (Aricept) for reducing the incidence of postoperative delirium after elective total hip replacement. Int J Geriatr Psychiatry 2007;22(4):343–9.
105. Leslie DL, Zhang Y, Bogardus ST, et al. Consequences of preventing delirium in hospitalized older adults on nursing home costs. J Am Geriatr Soc 2005;53(3):405–9.
106. Liptzin B, Levkoff SE. An empirical study of delirium subtypes. Br J Psychiatry 1992;161:843–5.
107. Inouye SK, Foreman MD, Mion LC, et al. Nurses' recognition of delirium and its symptoms. Comparison of nurse and researcher ratings. Arch Intern Med 2001;161(20):2467–73.
108. Stagno D, Gibson C, Breitbart W. The delirium subtypes: a review of prevalence, phenomenology, pathophysiology, and treatment response. Palliat Support Care 2004;2(2):171–9.
109. de Rooij SE, Schuurmans MJ, van der Mast RC, et al. Clinical subtypes of delirium and their relevance for daily clinical practice: a systematic review. Int J Geriatr Psychiatry 2005;20(7):609–15.

110. Marcantonio E, Ta T, Duthie E, et al. Delirium severity and psychomotor types: their relationship with outcomes after hip fracture repair. J Am Geriatr Soc 2002;50(5):850–7.
111. Santana Santos F, Wahlund LO, Varli F, et al. Incidence, clinical features and subtypes of delirium in elderly patients treated for hip fractures. Dement Geriatr Cogn Disord 2005;20(4):231–7.
112. American Psychiatric Association. Diagnostic and statistical manual of mental disorders, 4th edition. text revision (DSM-IV-TR). Washington, DC: American Psychiatric Association; 2000.
113. American Psychiatric Association. Practice guideline for the treatment of patients with delirium. Washington, DC: American Psychiatric Association; 1999.
114. Kikura M, Oikawa F, Yamamoto K, et al. Myocardial infarction and cerebrovascular accident following noncardiac surgery: differences in postoperative temporal distribution and risk factors. J Thromb Haemost 2008;6(5):742–8.
115. Stamou SC, Hill PC, Dangas G, et al. Stroke after coronary artery bypass: incidence, predictors, and clinical outcome. Stroke 2001;32(7):1508–13.
116. Ferro JM, Caeiro L, Verdelho A. Delirium in acute stroke. Curr Opin Neurol 2002;15(1):51–5.
117. Schuurmans MJ, Deschamps PI, Markham SW, et al. The measurement of delirium: review of scales. Res Theory Nurs Pract 2003;17(3):207–24.
118. Neelon VJ, Champagne MT, Carlson JR, et al. The NEECHAM Confusion Scale: construction, validation, and clinical testing. Nurse Res 1996;45(6): 324–30.
119. Gemert van LA, Schuurmans MJ. The NEECHAM confusion scale and the delirium observation screening scale: capacity to discriminate and ease of use in clinical practice. BMC Nurs 2007; 6:1–6.
120. Schuurmans MJ, Shortridge-Baggett LM, Duursma SA. The delirium observation screening scale: a screening instrument for delirium. Res Theory Nurs Pract 2003;17(1):31–50.
121. Inouye SK, van Dyck CH, Alessi CA, et al. Clarifying confusion: the confusion assessment method. A new method for detection of delirium. Ann Intern Med 1990;113(12):941–8.
122. Ely EW, Inouye SK, Bernard GR, et al. Delirium in mechanically ventilated patients: validity and reliability of the confusion assessment method for the intensive care unit (CAM-ICU). J Am Med Assoc 2001;286(21):2703–10.
123. Trzepacz PT, Mittal D, Torres R, et al. Validation of the Delirium Rating Scale-revised-98: comparison with the delirium rating scale and the cognitive test for delirium. J Neuropsychiatry Clin Neurosci 2001;13(2):229–42.
124. Boland RJ, Diaz S, Lamdan RM, et al. Overdiagnosis of depression in the general hospital. Gen Hosp Psychiatry 1996;18(1):28–35.
125. Rolfson DB, McElhaney JE, Jhangri GS, et al. Validity of the confusion assessment method in detecting postoperative delirium in the elderly. Int Psychogeriatr 1999;11(4):431–8.
126. Brauer C, Morrison RS, Silberzweig SB, et al. The cause of delirium in patients with hip fracture. Arch Intern Med 2000;160(12):1856–60.
127. Lonergan E, Britton AM, Luxenberg J. Antipsychotics for delirium. Cochrane Database Syst Rev 2007;(Issue 2). Art No: CD005594.
128. Bayindir O, Akpinar B, Can E, et al. The use of the 5-HT3-receptor antagonist ondansetron for the treatment of postcardiotomy delirium. J Cardiothorac Vasc Anesth 2000;14(3):288–92.
129. Heiser JF, Wilbert DE. Reversal of delirium induced by tricyclic antidepressant drugs with physostigmine. Am J Psychiatry 1974;131(11):1275–7.
130. Morita T, Akechi T, Ikenaga M, et al. Terminal delirium: recommendations from bereaved families' experiences. J Pain Symptom Manage 2007;34(6): 579–89.
131. Saliba D, Elliott M, Rubenstein LZ, et al. The vulnerable elders survey: a tool for identifying vulnerable older people in the community. J Am Geriatr Soc 2001;49(12):1691–9.
132. Assessing care of vulnerable elders-3 quality indicators. J Am Geriatr Soc 2007;55(Suppl 2): S464–87.

Chemotherapy in the Older Patient with Operable Non–Small Cell Lung Cancer: Neoadjuvant and Adjuvant Regimens

Ilene Browner, MD[a,b], Michael Purtell, MD, PhD[b,*]

KEYWORDS

- Non–small cell lung cancer • Elderly • Operable
- Adjuvant chemotherapy • Neoadjuvant chemotherapy

Lung cancer is the second most common form and the leading cause of cancer-related deaths in the United States. Non–small cell lung cancer (NSCLC) accounts for 85% of all incident lung cancer cases, and only 30% of these cases are diagnosed at an early stage.[1] Surgical resection is definitive therapy for early stage, especially node-negative, disease; however, overall survival is poor, with a 5-year survival rate of 15% for all stages and 55%, 45%, and 25% for completely resected stage I, II, and IIIA NSCLC, respectively.[2] Long-term survival for resected stage I-IIIA disease is compromised by a high rate of early distant and local recurrences attributed to the presence of micrometastatic disease not eradicated by surgery alone.[3] To improve survival outcomes and decrease disease recurrence postoperatively, strategies have been explored to improve surgical outcomes. These approaches include neoadjuvant/induction (preoperative) or adjuvant (postoperative) chemotherapy (with or without radiotherapy). Chemotherapy in both settings has afforded an absolute 5% benefit in overall survival;[4–6] however, the benefit of systemic therapy in older patients with NSCLC is not clearly defined.

Despite older adults being disproportionately affected by cancer, with 60% of all cancer diagnoses and 70% of all cancer-related deaths occurring in persons aged more than 65 years,[1] their enrollment in clinical trials woefully underrepresents their population numbers and cancer cases. Presently, about 6% of the population is 65 years of age or older; it is estimated that by the year 2030, 20% of the population will be in this age range.[7] With the rapid aging of America, the burden of cancer will only increase among the older population. This shift in burden is reflected in an increase in the mean age of incident cancers and, in particular, in lung cancer from 62 to 71 years of age. Additionally, 50% of lung cancers occur in persons 65 years of age or older, and lung cancer is the leading cause of cancer-related deaths among septuagenarians;[8] however, lung cancer–related mortality is decreasing among patients younger than 65 years. This discrepancy may be attributed to physiologic differences in the aged which impact tumor behavior, treatment tolerance and benefit, and differences in patterns of care.

Surgery, the mainstay of treatment for localized NSCLC, is safe and effective for older patients who are carefully selected based on a thorough preoperative assessment, including an estimate of life expectancy, function, polypharmacy, comorbid illnesses, and geriatric syndromes.[9,10] In a disease

[a] Division of Geriatric Medicine and Gerontology, Bayview Medical Center, Johns Hopkins Hospital, Baltimore, MD 21224, USA
[b] Department of Medical Oncology, Bayview Medical Center, Johns Hopkins Hospital, Baltimore, MD 21224, USA
* Corresponding author.
E-mail address: mpurtell@jhmi.edu (M. Purtell).

Thorac Surg Clin 19 (2009) 377–389
doi:10.1016/j.thorsurg.2009.07.005
1547-4127/09/$ – see front matter

thoracic.theclinics.com

that is fatal if not treated, surgery, irrespective of chronologic age but mindful of physiologic vulnerability, should be considered in early stage disease; however, there is a paucity of treatment and outcome data to guide decision making for this selected subgroup of older NSCLC patients.

Several excellent, non–age-specific review articles and meta-analyses have summarized in detail the available trials of surgery and either induction or adjuvant therapy with or without local radiotherapy in the treatment of early NSCLC.[5,6,11–13] A detailed review of the literature on the comprehensive assessment of and chemotherapy in elderly patients with NSCLC, which predominantly addresses inoperable, locally advanced, or metastatic disease, is beyond the scope of this article. Instead, the aim is to amalgamate the two topics and develop some practical guidelines to assist the clinician in deciding which therapies are appropriate for older patients.

EVALUATION OF THE OLDER CANCER PATIENT

Information on tumor and patient characteristics, the application of and benefit from therapy, and survival for older NSCLC patients is limited by their underenrollment in clinical trials.[14] Despite 60% of incident cancer cases occurring in patients aged older than 65 years, fewer than 25% of older adults participate in trials secondary to restrictive inclusion criteria, incomplete staging of disease, and age-related differences in patterns of care.[15] Underrepresentation in clinical trials limits knowledge of and evidence for treatment recommendations and benefit for older patients with cancer. Without evidence of benefit, many older patients are denied optimal therapy, with age as the primary barrier to care.[16,17] Among patients with NSCLC older than 80 years, only 30% are offered stage-specific, guideline-recommended therapy.[18] Extrapolation of data to older patients from trials assessing younger patients with NSCLC may lead to suboptimal therapy or harm. Trials for lung cancer have unintentionally excluded older persons from enrollment based on advanced age, increased burden of comorbid illness, and poorer performance status.

Chronologic age and its inherent physiologic changes have served as a barrier to care. Historically, age greater than 65 years has been used to define a person as "old"; however, with the aging of the population and the improvement in life expectancy due to better access to and advances in health care and sanitation, this arbitrary cut-off is no longer applicable as a definition of old age.[19] Physiologic age, a measure of fitness and functional reserve, may be a more reliable measure of global health and treatment tolerability among older patients. Assessment of fitness includes an estimate of vulnerability, life expectancy, functional status, polypharmacy, the burden and severity of comorbid illnesses, organ function, geriatric syndromes, and social and financial support. Collectively, this multidimensional definition of age is a more accurate reflection of an individual's tolerance of disease burden and treatment. Evaluation tools and their application to older cancer patients are being actively studied by experts in the field of geriatric oncology.[20–24] The American Society of Clinical Oncology, the International Society of Geriatric Oncology, and the National Comprehensive Cancer Network provide guidelines for the assessment of older patients with cancer.[25–27] Application of geriatric assessment techniques to the evaluation of the older cancer patient enhances the decision-making process concerning eligibility for local (surgery and radiation) and systemic therapies, and identifies previously undetected yet remediable issues in more than 30% of patients, leading to modifications in treatment planning and improved outcomes.[10,28,29]

INDUCTION AND ADJUVANT THERAPIES FOR EARLY STAGE NON–SMALL CELL LUNG CANCER

Overall survival for all stages of NSCLC is poor. Patients with early stage NSCLC fare better, but survival rates after curative surgical resection are suboptimal. Perioperative morbidity and mortality account, in part, for poor survival in this subset of patients, but, more frequently, distant and local recurrences are the most common cause of mortality.[30] Micrometastatic disease at the time of resection is the most likely source of relapsed disease. Neoadjuvant and adjuvant systemic and local therapies have been added to surgery as a means of addressing undetectable disease and reducing the relapse rate. Several randomized trials have demonstrated a modest, reproducible, absolute survival benefit for adjuvant therapy.[31] The impact of neoadjuvant therapy on survival is less well defined, but recent pooled analyses of small trials suggest a trend toward a survival benefit similar to that for adjuvant therapy.[6]

RATIONALE FOR NEOADJUVANT THERAPY IN NON–SMALL CELL LUNG CANCER

There are several theoretical advantages of administering therapy before surgery (**Box. 1**). The presumptive role of neoadjuvant therapy is to improve therapeutic benefit and, in turn, survival via early treatment of micrometastatic disease

Box 1
Theoretical advantages of neoadjuvant chemotherapy for non–small cell lung cancer

Superior distribution of chemotherapeutic agent to tumor

Early treatment of micrometastatic disease

Inhibition of inflammatory and growth factors

Direct assessment of tumor responsiveness to therapy

Calibration of fitness for surgery

Pre-operative downstaging of tumor

Reduction of perioperative stress

superior distribution of drug to the tumor, inhibition of tumoral inflammatory growth factors, and downstaging of tumor.[11,12] Micrometastatic disease has been detected by newer molecular techniques and is reflected in the high rate of distant recurrence after definitive surgical resection. Neoadjuvant treatment before surgical disruption of the vasculature may have a greater therapeutic benefit (distributing a higher volume of drug to the tumor) and may reduce the hematogenous spread of microscopic disease. Preoperative chemotherapy also may be better tolerated when administered before incurring the physiologic stresses associated with surgery, including the release of cytokines and growth factors during acute injury and recovery. This benefit may be of particular importance to older patients with a vulnerability to systemic stressors secondary to homeostatic fragility. The synergy of postsurgical inflammation with the overexpression of inflammatory cytokines associated with chronic illness and aging can destabilize compensated but fragile physiologic and functional reserves. A suitable response to neoadjuvant therapy also may downstage the tumor, allowing for a less extensive operation or a more complete resection.[32] In an older patient with borderline resection parameters such as decreased cardiac perfusion and contractility, diminished pulmonary function, and elevated pulmonary arterial pressure, or who would require a pneumonectomy, a good response to preoperative therapy may allow resection. Finally, a complete pathologic response to therapy predicts for improved survival.[33]

In addition to the survival benefit of neoadjuvant therapy, there are theoretical benefits as well. Inadequate treatment response, disease progression during neoadjuvant therapy, or poor tolerance for therapy may identify those patients for whom surgery may not be warranted, especially for patients considered to be borderline surgical candidates. Older patients who are more likely to have concurrent cardiovascular disease, chronic obstructive pulmonary disease, and a decreased pulmonary reserve (with a decreased diffusing capacity and thoracic compliance) may not have the physiologic reserves to tolerate both chemotherapy and surgery, especially if the chemotherapy follows the thoracotomy. Neoadjuvant therapy may serve as a litmus test for surgery and adjuvant therapies. Subgroup analyses of older patients who participated in adjuvant therapy trials for resectable NSCLC demonstrated poor tolerance for postoperative chemotherapy. Less than 50% of older patients as compared with nearly 80% of the younger patients received the planned number of treatment cycles.[34,35] Although a reduction in the total dose of chemotherapy did not appear to dilute the survival advantage of adjuvant chemotherapy, the long-term benefit may be affected. Neoadjuvant therapy may allow for (near) total delivery of planned cycles and thus, improved survival.

The primary disadvantage of neoadjuvant therapy is tumor resistance to the prescribed therapy and the possibility of disease progression, precluding the planned surgery or transitioning a patient from curable to incurable disease. In addition, the side effects of chemotherapy could further compromise a functionally borderline patient, delaying (or aborting) definitive surgery. Newer molecular diagnostic techniques that better characterize the host and the tumor, and ongoing neoadjuvant trials may help to individualize the treatment of early stage NSCLC, select patients appropriate for neoadjuvant therapy, and improve treatment outcomes.

The presumptive therapeutic role of neoadjuvant chemotherapy has been tested in several trials (**Table. 1**).[36–42] Many of the early trials were feasibility studies without a proper "surgery only" control group. Nevertheless, these studies suggested a survival advantage with neoadjuvant chemotherapy when compared with historical control groups. In the early 1990s, two studies comparing neoadjuvant chemotherapy followed by surgery with surgery alone in resectable stage IIIA disease demonstrated a statistically significant median survival benefit for the neoadjuvant arm.[38,39] The M.D. Anderson trial[39] randomized 60 patients to either cisplatin-based induction therapy or surgery alone. The preoperative chemotherapy group had an average survival at 3 years of 56% compared with a rate of 15% for those receiving surgery alone; this benefit has been maintained over time. Similarly, Rosell and colleagues[38] demonstrated a statistically significant survival

Table 1
Neoadjuvant trials for operable non–small cell lung cancer

Trial	Number of Patients	Stage	Regimen	Adherence	Response Rate	Survival (95% CI)
Rosell[38]	60	IIIA	MIC	—	—	HR, 0.63 (0.32–1.24)
Roth[39]	60	IIIA	CECy	—	—	HR, 0.89 (0.42–1.88)
Depierre[42]	355	IB-IIIA	MIC	90%	64% 11% pCR	HR, 0.83 (0.64–1.07) ~Median survival
BLOT[36]	94	IB-II	PC	96%	56% 6% pCR	—
SWOG 9990[37]	354	IB-II	PC	—	41%	~Median survival
MRC LU22/NVALT2/ EORTC 08,012[41]	519	IB-IIIa	GC, MIC, VC, MVC, DCar or PCar	91%	82.6% 5.3% pCR	HR, 1.02 (0.80–1.31) ~Progression-free survival
NATCH[40]	616	IA-IIIA	PC	—	—	—

Abbreviations: BLOT, Bimodality Lung Oncology Team; CE, cisplatin and etoposide; CECy, cisplatin, etoposide; DCar, docetaxel and carboplatin, cyclophosphamide; GC, gemcitabine and cisplatin; HR, hazard ratio of death; MIC, mitomycin C, ifosfamide, and cisplatin; MVC, mitomycin C, vinblastine, and cisplatin; NATCH, Neoadjuvant Taxol/Carboplatin Hope Trial; PC, paclitaxel and cisplatin; pCR, pathological complete response; PCar, paclitaxel and carboplatin; VC, vinorelbine and cisplatin.

benefit for the induction chemotherapy arm ($P<.001$), independent of the patient's age. Patients in this arm had a 10-month average survival, and there were no long-term survivors. In retrospect, the poor survival of the surgical group may reflect an imbalance of prognostic factors, with the surgery only group having more patients with K-RAS mutations.[43] In both trials, patients enrolled in the surgery only arm did not fare as well as expected based on other surgery only or clinical series. Therefore, the benefit of (neo) adjuvant chemotherapy may have been overestimated as a function of selection. The French Thoracic Cooperative Group trial[42] randomized 355 patients with stage I-IIIA disease to either surgery or preoperative chemotherapy with mitomycin C, ifosfamide, and cisplatin (MIC) followed by surgery. Stage I to III disease was included to address the suboptimal survival for early resected NSCLC. An overall, nonstatistically significant survival benefit was demonstrated for the neoadjuvant arm ($P = .15$), favoring patients with N0 and N1 disease (odds ratio, 0.68; $P = .027$). Recently, data from The Spanish Lung Cancer Group Trial 9901,[44] in which 136 patients were considered for induction chemotherapy with cisplatin, gemcitabine and docetaxel, reported those who were able to have a complete resection or had a clinical response to chemotherapy had a significant survival advantage ($P \leq .001$). In this trial, age less than 60 years was prognostic of a better outcome (hazard ratio [HR], 0.64; $P = .027$).

Small sample size, low statistical power, and the use of older, less well-tolerated chemotherapy regimens limit the ability to generalize the results of these trials to clinical and current practice. The Southwest Oncology Group (SWOG) 9900 trial[37] was designed to overcome some of these limitations through the accrual of a sufficient number of patients. Unfortunately, the trial was prematurely terminated when the positive results from adjuvant trials were reported, making postoperative chemotherapy the standard of care. Despite enrolling only 354 patients (half the planned accrual) with stage I-IIIA disease, the data favored the preoperative chemotherapy (paclitaxel and carboplatin) group for all stages by about 4% ($P = .47$). Although the LU22/NVALT2/EORTC 08,012 trial[41] (n = 519) did not demonstrate a significant survival benefit for neoadjuvant therapy (HR, 1.02; 95% CI, 0.8–1.31), it did report improvement in symptoms and downstaging of tumor in the neoadjuvant arm. Decreased symptoms and perhaps indirect improvement in survival reflected by tumor response and the likelihood of a complete resection may be of great importance to the older population that often favors quality over quantity of life (if the risk for toxicity and loss of function are high) and may be at greater risk for surgical morbidity and mortality.

Although the neoadjuvant arms showed better disease-free and overall survivals for most of these trials. The majority of the trials did not offer a statistically significant benefit favoring neoadjuvant over adjuvant therapy in the treatment of early stage, resectable NSCLC. Meta-analyses have been performed to overcome some of the limitations of each trial and to assess their collective impact on survival.[6,13] An estimated 6% overall survival benefit at 5 years for node-positive patients was calculated from the pooled results of these trials. This benefit is similar to the survival benefit demonstrated in a meta-analysis assessing the benefit of postoperative chemotherapy;[4] therefore, neoadjuvant therapy may be a reasonable treatment option in selected patients.

The role for and benefit of neoadjuvant therapy for older patients with early stage NSCLC are uncertain at best. Most of the neoadjuvant trials had an upper age limit of 75 years and did not include age-related data or subgroup analyses for the variable of age. Results from these trials cannot be directly extrapolated to the care of older NSCLC patients. Issues not clearly addressed by these trials, yet pertinent to the older patient, are age-specific pharmacokinetics of the selected agents, treatment toxicity as a function of physiologic age, and the disease-free and overall survival benefits of therapy. Although neoadjuvant regimens appear to be well tolerated by enrolled patients and the response rate to therapy appears to be independent of age, the tolerance for chemotherapy and the overall benefit among older patients, in comparison with younger patients, cannot be directly assessed.

In general, older patients gain "equal benefit from equal treatment"[45–47] when properly selected for and closely monitored during therapy; however, these data are from age-specific or age-inclusive trials of therapeutic regimens for stage IIIB and IV NSCLC but not for early stage disease.[14,48] In these trials, older patients had more pronounced renal and hepatic dysfunction, rendering them more likely to experience grade 3 or worse hematological and gastrointestinal treatment-related toxicities and to require more frequent dose modifications. Despite lower doses and fewer cycles of therapy administered in the palliative and neoadjuvant trials, response to therapy among older patients was similar to that among younger patients. In terms of specific regimens, there is a suggestion that the elderly may have increased toxicity with cisplatin as opposed to carboplatin[49–51] and that they may not benefit as much from multiple-drug regimens;[52] however, there are no active neoadjuvant trials assessing the toxicity and benefit of a carboplatin doublet or single-agent therapy.

Despite these constraints, patients aged more than 65 years would likely benefit in a fashion similar to younger patients if they fulfill the eligibility criteria of the trials. Currently, eligibility criteria for trials are becoming more inclusive with respect to age, performance status, and comorbidities; therefore, future NSCLC trials will likely better represent the evolving cancer demographic. Based on the current available evidence, if neoadjuvant therapy is to be considered in the elderly, the patient should be deemed fit enough to tolerate a platinum doublet, preferably a cisplatin-based regimen.

Lacking sufficient evidence for the role and benefit of neoadjuvant therapy among older patients with resectable NSCLC, preoperative therapy might be used to screen for those patients with aggressive or nonresponsive disease as well as patients with poor tolerance for or benefit from surgical intervention. Several studies have shown that patients with mediastinoscopy-confirmed N2 disease before neoadjuvant therapy, but with residual N2 disease at thoracotomy, fare significantly worse than those whose mediastinum is sterilized by the preoperative chemotherapy.[32,33,44,53,54] In INT 0139, patients eligible for enrollment had pathologically staged N2 nodes and were deemed "resectable." All of the patients received induction therapy with concurrent chemotherapy and radiation. Patients were randomized to additional radiation or to surgery. For the surgical arm, reexamination of the mediastinal nodes occurred at time of thoracotomy. The survival data showed that patients with a sterilized mediastinum at surgery had a 3-year survival rate of about 45% compared with 18% for patients with persistent nodal disease.[55] In patients with a node-positive mediastinoscopy after neoadjuvant chemotherapy, transition to definitive radiation rather than curative surgery may be warranted.

For technical reasons, it is difficult to perform two mediastinoscopies on the same patient. Less invasive methods, such as endoscopic bronchoscopy (EBUS) and positron emission tomography (PET) radioisotope imaging, can be employed to access the mediastinum. Pretherapy EBUS has about a 10% false-negative rate.[56] PET-CT imaging after chemotherapy or radiation has a sensitivity of about 70%, which is better than the results from a second mediastinoscopy.[57–59] In individuals for whom the immediate and long-term consequences of resection would not be warranted unless there was a reasonable chance for cure with surgery, an initial staging of the mediastinum via EBUS (with the sampling perhaps directed by a PET-CT) could be performed, preserving the use of the mediastinoscopy for use after induction therapy and before surgical resection. The converse order also would be reasonable, because EBUS can be used to restage the mediastinum after an initial mediastinoscopy.[56] Alternatively, after an initial staging mediastinoscopy and neoadjuvant therapy, one might reassess with PET-CT; however, the degree of false-positive and false-negative results might limit the usefulness of this approach.[60] For older patients, multimodality staging and risk stratification and neoadjuvant chemotherapy may be of greater consequence since this population is perceived as having the potential for increased morbidity and mortality with surgery. In addition, their actuarial predicted survival may be such that one may have reservations about subjecting them to surgery if they may not live sufficiently long enough to enjoy the presumed survival benefit of surgery vis a vis definitive radiation.

USE OF CHEMOTHERAPY BEFORE OR CONCURRENT WITH RADIATION

Clinical trials have been performed to assess the additive benefit of induction or concurrent chemotherapy to radiotherapy in patients with unresectable bulky N2 or N3 disease. Addition of chemotherapy was proposed given the poor median and 5-year survival with radiotherapy alone. The Cancer and Leukemia Group B (CALGB) 8433 trial randomized 155 patients with unresectable stage IIIA or IIIB NSCLC to radiation or induction chemotherapy with three cycles of cisplatin and vinblastine followed by radiation. After 7 years of follow-up, there was a sustained, significant median survival advantage for the induction arm when compared with the radiation arm (13.7 versus 9.6 months, $P = .012$).[61] In the phase III trial conducted by the Radiation Therapy Oncology Group (RTOG), Eastern Cooperative Oncology Group (ECOG), and SWOG, 458 patients with unresectable stage II-IIIB disease were randomized to radiation versus induction chemotherapy with cisplatin and vinblastine followed by radiation. A survival advantage was demonstrated for the induction chemotherapy arm.[62] Subsequently, RTOG 94-10 demonstrated that chemotherapy given concurrently with radiation was superior to a sequential schedule.[63] In both studies, subgroup analyses were performed on the variable of age greater or less than 70 years. In the sequential study, increases in chemotherapy-related mortality overwhelmed any survival benefit from the addition of chemotherapy. In the combined study, the older patients when compared with the younger patients appeared to benefit as much as if not more from the addition of chemotherapy despite increases in short-term side effects such as esophagitis.[50] The North Central Cancer Treatment Group 94-24-52 trial[64] was designed to assess cisplatin-etoposide chemotherapy concurrent with either daily or twice daily radiotherapy. A subanalysis of this trial examined the relationship between age and treatment outcome. The data demonstrated no differences in tumor progression or overall survival rates as a function of radiation schedule or age; however, grade 4 toxicity was more pronounced among patients aged 70 years or older (81% as compared with 62%, $P = .007$). The discrepancy between the two trials of concurrent therapy may reflect improvement in radiation techniques, differences in chemotherapy regimens, or patient selection. Data from two trials of induction chemotherapy followed by concurrent chemoradiation[65,66] suggest that such induction chemotherapy would likely add toxicity without providing sufficient benefit, limiting the utility of this regimen for most patients and, in particular, older patients. For fit older patients, concurrent chemoradiation is a viable treatment option; however, for patients deemed vulnerable to the vagaries of therapy, treatment with either the sequential protocol or radiation alone should be considered.

RATIONALE FOR ADJUVANT THERAPY IN NON–SMALL CELL LUNG CANCER

NSCLC has a poorer overall survival rate than other solid tumors and an approximately 50% likelihood of recurrence after complete resection of early stage disease. Poor outcomes in resected NSCLC may be attributable to micrometastatic disease at presentation.[67] The precedent for adjuvant therapy for NSCLC is set by effective adjuvant treatments for colon and breast cancer and the small but appreciable benefit of neoadjuvant therapy in NSCLC. Historically, trials designed to assess the benefit of adjuvant chemotherapy have been limited by a lack of statistical power, suboptimal and toxic chemotherapy regimens, and inconsistent staging of the mediastinum. When these studies were grouped in a meta-analysis published by the Non–Small Cell Lung Cancer Collaborative Group, their pooled data suggested a trend toward improved overall survival (HR, 0.87; 95%CI, 74–1.02) and an absolute survival benefit of 5% at 5 years with adjuvant cisplatin-based regimens.[4] Several larger randomized trials were initiated to confirm the benefit of adjuvant therapy for early stage NSCLC (**Table 2**).[68–75]

The Adjuvant Lung Project Italy (ALPI) trial randomized stage I-IIIA patients to surgery with observation or with mitomycin C/cisplatin/vindesine (MVP) chemotherapy. After 5 years of follow-up, there was no statistically significant difference in overall or progression-free survival between the two study arms.[72] Poor adherence to and significant toxicity from MVP suggested that a three-drug regimen might not be optimal in

Table 2
Adjuvant chemotherapy trials for resected early stage non–small cell lung cancer

Trial	Number of Patients	Stage	Regimen	Adherence	Toxicity	5-Year Survival (95% CI)
ALPI[72]	1088	I-IIIa	MVC	69%	12% grade 4 neutropenia	HR,0.96(0.81–1.13); *P* = .585
IALT[75]	1867	I-III	CE	73.8%	17.5% grade 4 neutropenia	HR, 0.86 (0.76–0.98); *P* <.03 4.1%
BLT[73]	381	I-III	VC, MIC, MVC, NC	>80%	30% grade 3/4 toxicity 3% deaths	HR,1.02(0.77–1.35); *P* = .9
ANITA01[70]	840	IB-IIIA	NC	>66%	85% grade 3/4 neutropenia 2% deaths	HR, 0.8 (0.66–0.96); *P* = .013 8.6%
JBR10[74]	482	IB-II	NC	—	—	HR, 0.69 (0.52–0.91); *P* = .04 15% at 2 years
CALGB 9633[71]	344	IB	PCar	86%	35% grade 3/4 neutropenia No deaths	HR, 0.80 (0.6-1.07) T≥4 cm HR, 0.69 (0.48–0.99)
UFT[69]	2000	I-II	UFT	—	—	HR, 0.71 (0.52–0.98) 6%

Abbreviations: ANITA, Adjuvant Navelbine International Trialist Association; ALPI, Adjuvant Lung Project Italy Trial; BLT, Big Lung Trial; CE, cisplatin and etoposide; HR, hazard ratio; IALT, International Adjuvant Lung Trial; JBR10, National Cancer Institute of Canada Intergroup trial; MIC, mitomycin C, ifosfamide, and cisplatin; MVC, mitomycin C, vinblastine, and cisplatin; NC, vinorelbine and cisplatin; PCar, paclitaxel and carboplatin; UFT, uracil-tegafur; VC, vindesine and cisplatin.

the adjuvant setting. On the other hand, the International Adjuvant Lung Trial (IALT), which randomized stage I-IIIA patients to postoperative observation or a cisplatin-based regimen, demonstrated a 4.1% absolute survival benefit associated with doublet adjuvant therapy ($P<.03$) at an average follow-up period of 56 months. Despite frequent grade 3 or 4 treatment-related toxicities and dose-reduced or incomplete delivery of planned therapy, patients at each stage benefited from cisplatin-based therapy; however, with an additional 3 years of follow up, this survival benefit was not sustained.[75] In like manner, the CALGB study 9633, which randomly assigned stage IB patients to adjuvant chemotherapy with paclitaxel and carboplatin or observation, initially suggested a survival benefit at 4 years for those receiving chemotherapy; however, at 74 months of follow-up, the survival benefit of adjuvant therapy when compared with observation was no longer evident (HR, 0.83; 90%CI, 0.64–1.08). A survival benefit for patients with tumors 4 cm or greater in diameter was demonstrated (HR, 0.69; 90%CI, 0.48–0.99).[71] The transient benefits seen in the IALT and CALGB 9633 trials may reflect any number of factors salient to the treatment of older cancer patients—the choice of cytotoxic agents and their late toxicity effects, the need for better definition of patient- and tumor-related prognostic markers, and the possible interactions among tumor, drug, and competing comorbid illness and functional status.[76] Additionally, the progression-free benefit, which is not altered by time, may be more important to older patients with a more limited life expectancy and a goal of prolonging life while maintaining their functional independence and global well-being.

Two other adjuvant studies firmly place cisplatin-based chemotherapy as the standard of care for postoperative treatment of patients with node-positive disease. The National Cancer Institute of Canada Intergroup JBR-10 trial randomized 482 patients with stage IB-II disease to postoperative cisplatin/vinorelbine or observation.[74] The 5-year absolute survival benefit of 15% favored the chemotherapy arm (HR, 0.69; 95%CI, 0.52–0.91) despite dose reductions and less than 50% adherence to all four planned treatment cycles. At 72 months, no benefit was seen for N0 patients, but there was an enduring 10% survival benefit for patients with N1 disease. Like the JBR10 trial, the Adjuvant Navelbine International Trialist Association (ANITA01) trial[70] showed a durable survival benefit for patients with positive hilar or mediastinal nodes treated with a cisplatin-based regimen;

node-negative patients did not benefit. The only data demonstrating a survival advantage for node-negative patients come from a meta-analysis of six randomized Japanese trials comparing surgery alone with 2 years of adjuvant uracil-tegafur (UFT) therapy.[69] Adjuvant UFT conferred a 7-year survival benefit of 7% among patients with stage IB but not IA tumors.[68] Similarly, six cycles of adjuvant cisplatin and etoposide significantly and durably improved disease-free and overall survival in stage IB patients with anatomic resection of their disease.[77]

Coming full circle, the Lung Adjuvant Cisplatin Evaluation (LACE) is a meta-analysis of pooled data from five of the cisplatin-based trials—the IALT, BIG, ANITA01, ALPI, and JBR10 trials.[5] LACE suggests that adjuvant cisplatin-based therapy improves overall survival by 5% to 10% in patients with N1 and N2 disease but not in patients with node-negative disease. The effect did not vary based on trial selected chemotherapy doublet; however, there was a trend toward additional benefit from the cisplatin-vinorelbine doublet (HR, 0.8; 95%CI, 0.7–0.91). Additionally, there was no interaction between age and chemotherapy effect, but there was a beneficial interaction between better performance status and treatment effect.[5] When considering cisplatin-based adjuvant chemotherapy, poor ECOG performance status (PS 2 or worse) may be a relative contraindication for prescription of adjuvant therapy.[78,79] This interaction is particularly pertinent to older patients with an increased frequency and severity of comorbid illnesses and greater vulnerability to physiologic stress.[80]

These trials are limited in their generalizability to the older population due to underenrollment or exclusion of patients with a high burden of comorbid illness, an ECOG PS greater than 1, or an age of 75 years or older. For the physician facing the decision of whether to offer adjuvant therapy to older patients, some age-specific data are available from subgroup analyses of the JBR-10 trial and LACE meta-analysis.[34,35] In the JBR-10 subanalysis, outcomes were compared among patients older (n = 155) and younger (n = 327) than 65 years; 23 patients were aged 75 years or older. Although older patients were much less likely to receive the planned number of cycles and the prescribed dose of therapy, chemotherapy prolonged their overall survival (HR, 0.61; 95%CI, 0.38–0.98), and the benefit was similar to the benefit for all patients treated in the JBR-10 trial (HR, 0.69; 95%CI, 0.52–0.91). There was no significant difference in treatment-related toxicity or death as a function of age.[35]

A subgroup analysis of the LACE meta-analysis of the variable of age on treatment outcomes reached a similar conclusion. There were no significant differences in cancer-related deaths, event-free survival, or rates of severe toxicity among patients aged more than 65 years (n = 1395), 65 to 69 years (n = 362), or 70 years or older (n = 157).[34] As in the JBR-10 trial, older patients received lower first and total cisplatin doses and fewer total chemotherapy cycles, but this dose reduction did not impact the beneficial treatment outcomes.

The age-dependent tendency toward dose reduction in both trials could not be explained wholly by trial design and may reflect the lack of evidenced-based data, the poorer performance status of the older patient population, or, indirectly, ageism in prescribing optimal treatment. Based on these results, age alone should not serve as a barrier to cisplatin-based chemotherapy for older patients with early stage, resected NSCLC; however, benefit from adjuvant therapy in older NSCLC patients will need to be demonstrated in prospective trials with more age-friendly inclusion criteria.

To date, the two trials with the most convincing results, JBR-10 and ANITA01, have employed an adjuvant regimen of cisplatin in combination with vinorelbine.[70,74] It is unclear whether the choice of chemotherapy regimen, patient selection, or other factors led to the trials' robust results. The current standard of care for patients with resected, node-positive, early stage NSCLC should be adjuvant therapy with cisplatin and vinorelbine; however, trepidation regarding the prescription of cisplatin-based therapy for the treatment of cancer in older adults is a viable concern. Some older patients with diminished physiologic and functional reserves, cardiovascular disease and other comorbidities, hearing loss, polypharmacy, drug- or disease-related neuropathy, and renal insufficiency may be more vulnerable to the well-documented toxic effects of and hydration for cisplatin therapy.

A retrospective analysis of ECOG 5592 was performed to compare outcomes of cisplatin-based doublet therapy for patients younger and older than 70 years with stage IIIB or IV disease and an ECOG PS of less than 2. Although the older subgroup had a higher burden of comorbid disease and treatment-related hematologic, cognitive, and nutritional toxicities, the response rate (P = .67), time to progression (P = .29), and survival (P = .29) were similar for older and younger patients.[50] Additionally, patients aged more than 80 years treated with cisplatin had stable renal function over time and no ototoxicity or neurotoxicity greater than or equal to grade 2; however, grade 3 or greater hematological and gastrointestinal toxicities were common.[49] Although cisplatin appears to be well tolerated in these retrospective analyses, the data cannot be directly extrapolated to clinical practice because age-specific, prospective data on pharmacokinetics and treatment effectiveness are not available. Cisplatin should not be used in older patients with borderline or pronounced renal dysfunction, and an estimated creatinine clearance should be calculated in all older patients even if the serum creatinine is normal.[81] Careful monitoring of renal function, volume status, auditory deficits, and neuropathy may limit adverse outcomes associated with delivery of cisplatin. Selection of older patients who are deemed fit to tolerate adjuvant therapy based on their perioperative health and recovery and their geriatric assessment and who have a predicted actuarial survival that would justify the risks (treatment toxicity) incurred from treatment would likely benefit from the small but undoubtedly real 5% to 10% advantage in predicted survival associated with cisplatin-based adjuvant therapy.[47]

FUTURE DIRECTIONS

Recent advances in the molecular biology of lung cancer will allow tailoring of therapies to the unique characteristics of hosts and their tumors. In the Rosell and colleagues[38] neoadjuvant and the JBR-10 adjuvant[74] studies, analyses of tumors for K-RAS mutation suggested that the presence of the mutation blunts or negates the benefit of adjuvant or neoadjuvant therapy. Although cisplatin-based therapy is supported by the trial data presented previously, patients whose tumor can subrogate the DNA damage through overexpression of the excision repair cross-complementation group-1 (ERCC1), an enzyme that assists in the repair of cisplatin-induced DNA damage, may not benefit from cisplatin therapy.[82] In addition, patients with higher levels of repair mechanisms have a better natural survival than those without.[83] Older patients with K-RAS mutations or increased ERCC1 activity may not sufficiently benefit from cisplatin-based neoadjuvant or adjuvant therapy to warrant its use. Whether these changes are expressed more frequently in older patients with NSCLC is unknown; however, decisions regarding cisplatin-based therapy may be guided by their expression until additional data are available, especially if the patient is assessed as being vulnerable to frail before or during therapy.

Mutations near the ATPase pocket of the EGFR1 receptor can render tumors sensitive to the antiproliferative effect of certain tyrosine kinase inhibitors (TKIs)[84] and may be a predictor of a longer time to treatment failure in advanced (and perhaps early) disease. Ongoing trials such as the Radiant trial[85] are assessing the role of TKIs as induction or adjuvant therapy for resectable NSCLC. Because TKIs are deemed less toxic than chemotherapy among older cancer patients,[16] they may be an appropriate alternative therapy for frailer patients with certain tumor characteristics.

Although the current data from (neo)adjuvant studies support the use of cisplatin-based regimens in early stage resectable NSCLC, it is unclear whether single or multi-agent regimens will have similar or superior efficacy and tolerability in the older patient. The current (Neo)Adjuvant Taxol/Carboplatin Hope (NATCH) trial, comparing three cycles of carboplatin and paclitaxel before or after surgery with surgery alone, will help define the role of and regimen for (neo)adjuvant chemotherapy for stages IA (T >2 cm) and IB-IIIA (T3N1) disease. Additionally, DNA markers will be evaluated to identify prognostic factors and markers of chemoresistance.[40] A recent report on the differential response of squamous carcinoma and adenocarcinoma to gemcitabine and pemetrexed may eventually prove useful in the selection of a more robust, possibly less toxic individualized treatment regimen.[86] Bevacizumab, an antibody to VEGFA ligand, has been shown to potentiate the response of carboplatin in combination with either paclitaxel or pemetrexed for advanced NSCLC.[87] The current E1505 adjuvant study is testing the hypothesis that this benefit can be replicated in the adjuvant setting; however, in older patients with advanced NSCLC, the addition of bevacizumab to palliative chemotherapy with paclitaxel and carboplatin has resulted in increased toxicity without improvement in survival.[88] The ANITA02 trial is an adjuvant study evaluating the therapeutic benefit of single agent vinorelbine. If this trial demonstrates equivalent or superior survival benefit with a single agent as compared to multiple drug regimens, the results may benefit older vulnerable to frail patients or those with reduced tolerance for multi-drug or cisplatin-based regimens. There are also emerging data that men may respond to and benefit from therapy differently than women; men benefit more from bevacizumab-based therapy whereas nonsmoking women benefit from treatment with TKIs. This perceived effect may be valuable in customizing treatment for the older patient.

SUMMARY

Whether a patient should receive systemic therapy before or after definitive surgical or radiation therapy is unclear because the survival benefit is only 5% to 10%, but, in certain cases, the physical and economic costs of therapy may far outweigh the benefit. The task at hand is to apply these data to the older NSCLC patient. For certain individuals with significant comorbid illnesses or limited life expectancy, disease-free survival and improved quality of life must be weighed against the possible treatment-related burden needed to realize the demonstrated survival benefit of (neo) adjuvant chemotherapy. For fit patients with resectable NSCLC and a life expectancy of greater than 2 years, such therapies should be considered even though elderly patients may suffer increased but tolerable toxicity from chemotherapy, radiation, and surgery. At present, neoadjuvant therapy might be prescribed for older patients who are deemed borderline for curative surgery, who would benefit from tumor downstaging, or who would be best served with definitive radiation if the neoadjuvant response was suboptimal. As these and other insights are clarified and supported by trial-based evidence, the physician may be better able to tailor therapies to improve treatment outcomes and limit toxicity among all patients and, in particular, older patients.

REFERENCES

1. Jemal A, Siegel R, Ward E, et al. Cancer statistics. CA Cancer J Clin 2008;58(2):71–96.
2. Nesbitt JC, Putnam JB Jr, Walsh GL, et al. Survival in early-stage non–small cell lung cancer. Ann Thorac Surg 1995;60(2):466–72.
3. Ou SH, Zell JA, Ziogas A, et al. Prognostic factors for survival of stage I non–small cell lung cancer patients: a population-based analysis of 19,702 stage I patients in the California cancer registry from 1989 to 2003. Cancer 2007;110(7):1532–41.
4. Non–Small Cell Lung Cancer Collaborative Group. Chemotherapy in non –small cell lung cancer: a meta-analysis using updated data on individual patients from 52 randomised clinical trials. Non–small cell lung cancer collaborative group. BMJ 1995;311(7010):899–909.
5. Pignon JP, Tribodet H, Scagliotti GV, et al. Lung adjuvant cisplatin evaluation: a pooled analysis by the LACE collaborative group. J Clin Oncol 2008;26(21):3552–9.
6. Berghmans T, Paesmans M, Meert AP, et al. Survival improvement in resectable non–small cell lung cancer with (neo)adjuvant chemotherapy: results of a meta-analysis of the literature. Lung Cancer 2005;49(1):13–23.
7. Aging statistics. Available at: http://www.aoa.gov/AoARoot/Aging_Statistics/index.aspx. Accessed June 13, 2009.
8. Rocha Lima CM, Herndon JE 2nd, Kosty M, et al. Therapy choices among older patients with lung carcinoma: an evaluation of two trials of the cancer and leukemia group B. Cancer 2002;94(1):181–7.
9. Spaggiari L, Scanagatta P. Surgery of non–small ce lung cancer in the elderly. Curr Opin Oncol 2007 19(2):84–91.
10. PACE participants, Audisio RA, Pope D, et al. Sha we operate? Preoperative assessment in elderl cancer patients (PACE) can help. A SIOG surgica task force prospective study. Crit Rev Oncol Hema tol 2008;65(2):156–63.
11. Belani CP. Adjuvant and neoadjuvant therapy i non–small cell lung cancer. Semin Oncol 2005;32(Suppl 2):S9–15.
12. Brahmer JR, Ettinger DS. Non–small cell lun cancer: adjuvant and neoadjuvant chemotherapy Respirology 2007;12(3):320–5.
13. Burdett S, Stewart LA, Rydzewska L. A systemati review and meta-analysis of the literature: chemo therapy and surgery versus surgery alone in non small cell lung cancer. J Thorac Oncol 2006;1(7) 611–21.
14. Vora N, Reckamp KL. Non–small cell lung cancer i the elderly: defining treatment options. Semin Onco 2008;35(6):590–6.
15. Peake MD, Thompson S, Lowe D, et al. Ageism i the management of lung cancer. Age Agein 2003;32(2):171–7.
16. Owonikoko TK, Ragin CC, Belani CP, et al. Lun cancer in elderly patients: an analysis of the survei lance, epidemiology, and end results database J Clin Oncol 2007;25(35):5570–7.
17. Smith TJ, Penberthy L, Desch CE, et al. Differences i initial treatment patterns and outcomes of lung cance in the elderly. Lung Cancer 1995;13(3):235–52.
18. Oxnard GR, Fidias P, Muzikansky A, et al. Non–sma cell lung cancer in octogenarians: treatment prac tices and preferences. J Thorac Oncol 2007;2(11) 1029–35.
19. Hurria A, Kris MG. Management of lung cancer i older adults. CA Cancer J Clin 2003;53(6):325–41.
20. Extermann M, Hurria A. Comprehensive geriatri assessment for older patients with cancer. J Cli Oncol 2007;25(14):1824–31.
21. Rodin MB, Mohile SG. A practical approach to ger atric assessment in oncology. J Clin Oncol 2007 25(14):1936–44.
22. Hurria A. Incorporation of geriatric principles i oncology clinical trials. J Clin Oncol 2007;25(34) 5350–1.
23. Hurria A, Lichtman SM, Gardes J, et al. Identifyin vulnerable older adults with cancer: integrating ger atric assessment into oncology practice. J Am Ge iatr Soc 2007;55(10):1604–8.
24. Klepin H, Mohile S, Hurria A. Geriatric assessment i older patients with breast cancer. J Natl Comp Canc Netw 2009;7(2):226–36.
25. Geriatric oncology: ASCO cancer portals. Available a http://geriatricsca.asco.org/CancerPortals/Geriatric-Oncology. Accessed June 13, 2009.

26. Geriatric assessment tools. Available at: http://www.siog.org/index.php?option=com_content&view=article&id=103&Itemid=78. Accessed June 13, 2009.
27. NCCN clinical practice guidelines in oncology: senior adult oncology. Available at: http://www.nccn.org/professionals/physician_gls/PDF/senior.pdf. Accessed June 13, 2009.
28. Cudennec T, Gendry T, Labrune S, et al. Use of a simplified geriatric evaluation in thoracic oncology. Lung Cancer 2009;64(Suppl 1):S72–3.
29. Girre V, Falcou MC, Gisselbrecht M, et al. Does a geriatric oncology consultation modify the cancer treatment plan for elderly patients? J Gerontol A Biol Sci Med Sci 2008;63(7):724–30.
30. Detterbeck FC, Socinski MA, Gralla RJ, et al. Neoadjuvant chemotherapy with gemcitabine-containing regimens in patients with early-stage non–small cell lung cancer. J Thorac Oncol 2008;3(1):37–45.
31. Alam N, Darling G, Evans WK, et al. Lung cancer disease site group of cancer care ontario's program in evidence-based care. Adjuvant chemotherapy for completely resected non–small cell lung cancer: a systematic review. Crit Rev Oncol Hematol 2006; 58(2):146–55.
32. D'Angelillo RM, Trodella L, Ramella S. Assessing the value of neoadjuvant chemoradiotherapy and pathologic downstaging in the treatment of non–small cell lung cancer. J Thorac Cardiovasc Surg 2004;128(3): 489–90.
33. Betticher DC, Hsu Schmitz SF, Totsch M, et al. Prognostic factors affecting long-term outcomes in patients with resected stage IIIA pN2 non–small cell lung cancer: 5-year follow-up of a phase II study. Br J Cancer 2006;94(8):1099–106.
34. Fruh M, Rolland E, Pignon JP, et al. Pooled analysis of the effect of age on adjuvant cisplatin-based chemotherapy for completely resected non–small cell lung cancer. J Clin Oncol 2008;26(21): 3573–81.
35. Pepe C, Hasan B, Winton TL, et al. Adjuvant vinorelbine and cisplatin in elderly patients: National Cancer Institute of Canada and Intergroup study JBR.10. J Clin Oncol 2007;25(12):1553–61.
36. Pisters KM, Ginsberg RJ, Giroux DJ, et al. Induction chemotherapy before surgery for early-stage lung cancer: a novel approach. Bimodality Lung Oncology Team. J Thorac Cardiovasc Surg 2000; 119(3):429–39.
37. Pisters K, Vallieres E, Bunn P, et al. S9900: a phase III trial of surgery alone or surgery plus preoperative (preop) paclitaxel/carboplatin (PC) chemotherapy in early stage non–small cell lung cancer (NSCLC). Preliminary results [abstract]. J Clin Oncol 2005; 23(16):LBA7012. Accessed June 13, 2009.
38. Rosell R, Gomez-Codina J, Camps C, et al. A randomized trial comparing preoperative chemotherapy plus surgery with surgery alone in patients with non–small cell lung cancer. N Engl J Med 1994;330(3):153–8.
39. Roth JA, Fossella F, Komaki R, et al. A randomized trial comparing perioperative chemotherapy and surgery with surgery alone in resectable stage IIIA non–small cell lung cancer. J Natl Cancer Inst 1994;86(9):673–80.
40. Felip E, Rosell R, Massuti B, et al. The NATCH trial: observations on the neoadjuvant arm [abstract]. J Clin Oncol 2007;25(18):7578.
41. Gilligan D, Nicolson M, Smith I, et al. Preoperative chemotherapy in patients with resectable non–small cell lung cancer: results of the MRC LU22/NVALT 2/EORTC 08012 multicentre randomised trial and update of systematic review. Lancet 2007; 369(9577):1929–37.
42. Depierre A, Milleron B, Moro-Sibilot D, et al. Preoperative chemotherapy followed by surgery compared with primary surgery in resectable stage I (except T1N0), II, and IIIa non–small cell lung cancer. J Clin Oncol 2002;20(1):247–53.
43. Rosell R, Felip E, Maestre J, et al. The role of chemotherapy in early non–small cell lung cancer management. Lung Cancer 2001;34(Suppl 3):S63–74.
44. Garrido P, Gonzalez-Larriba JL, Insa A, et al. Long-term survival associated with complete resection after induction chemotherapy in stage IIIA (N2) and IIIB (T4N0-1) non–small cell lung cancer patients: the Spanish Lung Cancer Group trial 9901. J Clin Oncol 2007;25(30):4736–42.
45. Balducci L. The geriatric cancer patient: equal benefit from equal treatment. Cancer Control 2001; 8(2 Suppl):27–8 [quiz: 1–25].
46. Gridelli C, Langer C, Maione P, et al. Lung cancer in the elderly. J Clin Oncol 2007;25(14):1898–907.
47. Gridelli C, Maione P, Comunale D, et al. Adjuvant chemotherapy in elderly patients with non–small cell lung cancer. Cancer Control 2007;14(1):57–62.
48. Gridelli C, Maione P, Rossi A, et al. Treatment of locally advanced non–small cell lung cancer in the elderly. Curr Opin Oncol 2005;17(2):130–4.
49. Thyss A, Saudes L, Otto J, et al. Renal tolerance of cisplatin in patients more than 80 years old. J Clin Oncol 1994;12(10):2121–5.
50. Langer CJ, Manola J, Bernardo P, et al. Cisplatin-based therapy for elderly patients with advanced non–small cell lung cancer: implications of Eastern Cooperative Oncology Group 5592, a randomized trial. J Natl Cancer Inst 2002;94(3):173–81.
51. Kubota K, Furuse K, Kawahara M, et al. Cisplatin-based combination chemotherapy for elderly patients with non–small cell lung cancer. Cancer Chemother Pharmacol 1997;40(6):469–74.
52. Frasci G, Southern Italy Cooperative Oncology Group (SICOG). Chemotherapy of lung cancer in the elderly. Crit Rev Oncol Hematol 2002;41(3):349–61.

53. Martini N, Kris MG, Flehinger BJ, et al. Preoperative chemotherapy for stage IIIa (N2) lung cancer: the Sloan-Kettering experience with 136 patients. Ann Thorac Surg 1993;55(6):1373–4 [discussion: 1365–73].
54. Takeda S, Maeda H, Okada T, et al. Results of pulmonary resection following neoadjuvant therapy for locally advanced (IIIA-IIIB) lung cancer. Eur J Cardiothorac Surg 2006;30(1):184–9.
55. Albain KS, Swann RS, Rusch VW, et al. Radiotherapy plus chemotherapy with or without surgical resection for stage III non-small-cell lung cancer: a phase III randomised controlled trial. Lancet 2009;374:379–86.
56. Herth FJ, Annema JT, Eberhardt R, et al. Endobronchial ultrasound with transbronchial needle aspiration for restaging the mediastinum in lung cancer. J Clin Oncol 2008;26(20):3346–50.
57. Eschmann SM, Friedel G, Paulsen F, et al. Repeat 18F-FDG PET for monitoring neoadjuvant chemotherapy in patients with stage III non–small cell lung cancer. Lung Cancer 2007;55(2):165–71.
58. De Leyn P, Stroobants S, De Wever W, et al. Prospective comparative study of integrated positron emission tomography–computed tomography scan compared with remediastinoscopy in the assessment of residual mediastinal lymph node disease after induction chemotherapy for mediastinoscopy-proven stage IIIA-N2 non–small cell lung cancer: a leuven lung cancer group study. J Clin Oncol 2006;24(21):3333–9.
59. Dooms C, Vansteenkiste J. Positron emission tomography in non–small cell lung cancer. Curr Opin Pulm Med 2007;13(4):256–60.
60. Tanvetyanon T, Eikman EA, Sommers E, et al. Computed tomography response, but not positron emission tomography scan response, predicts survival after neoadjuvant chemotherapy for resectable non–small cell lung cancer. J Clin Oncol 2008;26(28):4610–6.
61. Dillman RO, Herndon J, Seagren SL, et al. Improved survival in stage III non–small cell lung cancer: seven-year follow-up of cancer and leukemia Group B (CALGB) 8433 trial. J Natl Cancer Inst 1996;88(17):1210–5.
62. Sause W, Kolesar P, Taylor SIV, et al. Final results of phase III trial in regionally advanced unresectable non–small cell lung cancer: Radiation Therapy Oncology Group, Eastern Cooperative Oncology Group, and Southwest Oncology Group. Chest 2000;117(2):358–64.
63. Langer CJ, Hsu C, Curran W, et al. Do elderly patients with locally advanced non–small cell lung cancer (NSCLC) benefit from combined modality therapy? A secondary analysis of RTOG 94-10. Int J Radiat Oncol Biol Phys 2001;51(3):20–1.
64. Schild SE, Stella PJ, Geyer SM, et al. The outcome of combined-modality therapy for stage III non–small cell lung cancer in the elderly. J Clin Oncol 2003;21(17):3201–6.
65. Vokes EE, Herndon JE 2nd, Kelley MJ, et al. Induction chemotherapy followed by chemoradiotherapy compared with chemoradiotherapy alone for regionally advanced unresectable stage III non–small cell lung cancer: cancer and leukemia group B. J Clin Oncol 2007;25(13):1698–704.
66. Belani CP, Choy H, Bonomi P, et al. Combined chemoradiotherapy regimens of paclitaxel and carboplatin for locally advanced non–small cell lung cancer: a randomized phase II locally advanced multimodality protocol. J Clin Oncol 2005;23(25):5883–91.
67. Solomon B, Bunn PA Jr. Adjuvant chemotherapy for non–small cell lung cancer. Cancer Invest 2007;25(4):217–25.
68. Kato H, Ichinose Y, Ohta M, et al. A randomized trial of adjuvant chemotherapy with uracil-tegafur for adenocarcinoma of the lung. N Engl J Med 2004;350(17):1713–21.
69. Hamada C, Tanaka F, Ohta M, et al. Meta-analysis of postoperative adjuvant chemotherapy with tegafur-uracil in non–small cell lung cancer. J Clin Oncol 2005;23(22):4999–5006.
70. Douillard JY, Rosell R, De Lena M, et al. Adjuvant vinorelbine plus cisplatin versus observation in patients with completely resected stage IB-IIIA non–small cell lung cancer (Adjuvant Navelbine International Trialist Association [ANITA]): a randomised controlled trial. Lancet Oncol 2006;7(9):719–27.
71. Strauss GM, Herndon JE 2nd, Maddaus MA, et al. Adjuvant paclitaxel plus carboplatin compared with observation in stage IB non–small cell lung cancer: CALGB 9633 with the cancer and leukemia Group B, Radiation Therapy Oncology Group, and North Central Cancer Treatment Group study groups. J Clin Oncol 2008;26(31):5043–51.
72. Scagliotti GV. The ALPI trial: the Italian/European experience with adjuvant chemotherapy in resectable non–small lung cancer. Clin Cancer Res 2005;11(13 Pt 2):5011s–6s.
73. Waller D, Peake MD, Stephens RJ, et al. Chemotherapy for patients with non–small cell lung cancer: the surgical setting of the big lung trial. Eur J Cardiothorac Surg 2004;26(1):173–82.
74. Winton T, Livingston R, Johnson D, et al. Vinorelbine plus cisplatin versus observation in resected non–small cell lung cancer. N Engl J Med 2005;352(25):2589–97.
75. Le Chevalier T, Dunant A, Arriagada R, et al. Long-term results of the International Adjuvant Lung Cancer Trial (IALT) evaluating adjuvant cisplatin-based chemotherapy in resected non–small cell lung cancer (NSCLC) [abstract]. J Clin Oncol 2008;26(15):7507.
76. Besse B, Le Chevalier T. Adjuvant chemotherapy for non–small cell lung cancer: a fading effect? J Clin Oncol 2008;26(31):5014–7.

77. Roselli M, Mariotti S, Ferroni P, et al. Postsurgical chemotherapy in stage IB non–small cell lung cancer: long-term survival in a randomized study. Int J Cancer 2006;119(4):955–60.
78. Lee D. Benefit of active treatment in non–small cell lung cancer in elderly patients and patients with poor performance status. Clin Lung Cancer 2003;5(2):86–9.
79. Extermann M, Overcash J, Lyman GH, et al. Comorbidity and functional status are independent in older cancer patients. J Clin Oncol 1998;16(4):1582–7.
80. Janssen-Heijnen ML, Smulders S, Lemmens VE, et al. Effect of comorbidity on the treatment and prognosis of elderly patients with non–small cell lung cancer. Thorax 2004;59(7):602–7.
81. Lichtman SM, Wildiers H, Chatelut E, et al. International Society of Geriatric Oncology Chemotherapy Taskforce: evaluation of chemotherapy in older patients–an analysis of the medical literature. J Clin Oncol 2007;25(14):1832–43.
82. Olaussen KA, Dunant A, Fouret P, et al. DNA repair by ERCC1 in non–small cell lung cancer and cisplatin-based adjuvant chemotherapy. N Engl J Med 2006;355(10):983–91.
83. Zheng Z, Chen T, Li X, et al. DNA synthesis and repair genes RRM1 and ERCC1 in lung cancer. N Engl J Med 2007;356(8):800–8.
84. Yang CH, Yu CJ, Shih JY, et al. Specific EGFR mutations predict treatment outcome of stage IIIB/IV patients with chemotherapy-naive non–small cell lung cancer receiving first-line gefitinib monotherapy. J Clin Oncol 2008;26(16):2745–53.
85. Richardson F, Richardson K, Sennello D. Biomarker analysis from completely resected NSCLC patients enrolled in an adjuvant erlotinib clinical trial (RADIANT). J Clin Oncol 27: 15s. Available from: http://www.asco.org/ASCOv2/Meetings/Abstracts?&vmview=abst_detail_view&confID=60&abstractID=50126. Accessed July 10, 2009.
86. Scagliotti GV, Parikh P, von Pawel J, et al. Phase III study comparing cisplatin plus gemcitabine with cisplatin plus pemetrexed in chemotherapy-naive patients with advanced-stage non–small cell lung cancer. J Clin Oncol 2008;26(21):3543–51.
87. Sandler A, Gray R, Perry MC, et al. Paclitaxel-carboplatin alone or with bevacizumab for non-small-cell lung cancer. N Engl J Med 2006;355:2542–50.
88. Ramalingam SS, Dahlberg SE, Langer CJ, et al. Outcomes for elderly, advanced-stage non–small cell lung cancer patients treated with bevacizumab in combination with carboplatin and paclitaxel: analysis of Eastern Cooperative Oncology Group trial 4599. J Clin Oncol 2008;26(1):60–5.

Thoracic Irradiation in the Elderly

Kristin J. Redmond, MD, Danny Y. Song, MD*

KEYWORDS

- Lung cancer • Elderly • Thoracic irradiation
- Toxicity • Technology

The management of elderly patients with lung cancer is a growing problem. The median age at diagnosis of lung cancer is 70 years,[1] and more than half of the patients diagnosed with advanced non–small cell lung cancer (NSCLC) are greater than 65 years.[3] During the past decade the incidence and mortality from lung cancer has declined in patients younger than age 50 years but has increased in patients older than age 70 years.[4] Lung cancer diagnoses in elderly patients are expected to continue to increase during the next 20 years as the proportion of Americans over the age of 65 years rises, but it remains unclear whether standard therapy for lung cancer is appropriate in this patient population.

Oncologic care of elderly patients often is complicated by poor baseline performance status and medical comorbidities. Zeber and colleagues[5] recently reviewed the prevalence of comorbid conditions in patients greater than age 70 years diagnosed with lung, colorectal, prostate, or head and neck cancer at the Veterans Health Administration and found than 70% of their cohort had hypertension, more than 50% had hyperlipidemia, 40% had heart disease, 25% had diabetes, and 17% met criteria for frailty. These pre-existing conditions play an important role in treatment decisions, because they limit the elderly patient's ability to tolerate particular therapeutic options. Another consideration is that advanced age itself may contribute to a worse outcome in patients who have lung cancer. Recusive partitioning analyses of large databases by the European Lung Cancer Working Party, the Southwest Oncology Group, and the Radiation Therapy Oncology Group (ROTG) have found advanced age to be independently prognostic of survival.[6–8]

Data regarding the optimal therapy for elderly patients who have lung cancer are limited. There are very few randomized, controlled trials designed specifically for the elderly, and many of the phase III studies that guide standard therapy excluded patients over the age of 70 years. Even when elderly patients are not explicitly ineligible, the potential for selection bias persists, and because only fit elderly patients are likely to be enrolled in age-unspecified trials, it is difficult to extrapolate these data to the elderly population as a whole. Numerous questions regarding treatment of lung cancer in elderly patients remain. For example, if radiation to elderly patients results in increased toxicity, will the survival benefit decrease as a result of higher morbidity and mortality or decreased compliance? Would modified fractionation schedules be beneficial? These important questions will be answered effectively only by randomized clinical trials designed specifically for elderly patients. The North Central Cancer Treatment Group conducted a pooled analysis of elderly patients who participated in elderly-specific trials compared with age-unspecified trials and reported that elderly specific trials had a higher median age as well as lower rates of severe adverse events with no difference in survival.[9] This finding suggests that elderly-specific trials are critical in evaluating safe and effective therapies for this select patient population.

This article reviews thoracic irradiation in elderly patients. Specifically, it begins by discussing the role of radiation therapy in the management of lung cancer, regardless of age. It then examines the toxicity associated with the radiation therapy, which may be particularly problematic in elderly patients. Finally, it outlines radiotherapeutic

Department of Radiation Oncology and Molecular Radiation Sciences, The Johns Hopkins University School of Medicine, 401 North Broadway, Suite 1440, Baltimore, MD 21231, USA
* Corresponding author.
E-mail address: dsong2@jhmi.edu (D.Y. Song).

Thorac Surg Clin 19 (2009) 391–400
doi:10.1016/j.thorsurg.2009.06.003
1547-4127/09/$ – see front matter

thoracic.theclinics.com

methods that may be used to limit this toxicity so that elderly patients may be more likely to benefit from radiation therapy.

RADIATION THERAPY FOR LUNG CANCER

The use of radiation therapy for lung cancer depends on a variety of factors, such as histology, stage, and resectability of the tumor. The age of the patient does not directly guide therapy, but medical comorbidities are prevalent in elderly patients and may alter the type of treatments are available to them. This section reviews the role of radiation therapy in lung cancer, based on the histology and stage of disease, and examines the applicability of current evidence to elderly patients.

NSCLC

Early-stage disease

Therapy for NSCLC is stratified according to stage, either early or locally advanced. When safely feasible, surgical resection is the standard of care in early-stage disease. Unfortunately, as discussed earlier in this article, elderly patients are at higher risk than younger patients of medical comorbidities and frailty and have an increased likelihood of being deemed medically inoperable in spite of early-stage disease. Involved field radiation therapy (IFRT) encompasses pathologically or radiographically documented areas of disease involvement and is the standard treatment modality in patients who have inoperable stage I and stage II NSCLC.[10–13] Retrospective data suggest that outcomes after IFRT in medically inoperable elderly patients who have early-stage disease are comparable to those in younger patients. The same studies suggest that toxicity is acceptable, although slightly higher than in younger patients.[14,15] A small prospective phase I/II trial of IFRT using intensity-modulated radiation therapy in patients aged 70 years or older revealed an objective response rate of 88.6% with 1-, 2-, and 5-year overall survival rates of 65.8%, 55.7%, and 25.3%, respectively. Local progression-free survival was 84.8%, and toxicity was minimal, suggesting that IFRT is a reasonable option in elderly patients who have medically inoperable early-stage NSCLC.[16]

Locally advanced disease

Based on the results of several randomized clinical trials, the standard of care in patients who have unresectable advanced-stage NSCLC is concurrent radiation therapy and cisplatin-based chemotherapy.[17–20] Although the studies unequivocally favor concurrent chemoradiation, patients who have advanced age, poor Karnofsky performance status, or medical comorbidities generally were excluded from enrollment. As a result, the mean age of patients in these trials ranged from 54 to 63 years,[21] and the applicability of these results to elderly patients is unclear.

There are limited prospective data regarding the role of concurrent chemoradiation therapy in elderly patients who have locally advanced NSCLC. Phase II studies have demonstrated acceptable side-effect profiles, but the overall survival rates have been lower than in other trials. The median survival has ranged from 10 to 13 months in the elderly-specific studies versus 16 to 17 months in other studies.[22–25]

The Japanese Clinical Oncology Group performed a phase III trial in patients older than 70 years who had stage III NSCLC[26] in which patients were assigned randomly to radiation alone or to radiation plus concurrent daily carboplatin. Four deaths (one in the radiation-alone arm and three in the chemoradiation arm) led to premature closure of the study. Review of protocol compliance revealed that only 40% of radiation fields met specifications regarding tumor coverage or normal lung dose constraints. Furthermore, two of the four deaths occurred in conjunction with protocol violations regarding radiation fields, which were supposed to have been restricted to cover less than half of one lung. Because of the premature termination of the trial, only 46 patients were enrolled. Median survival was 14.3 months with radiation alone versus 18.5 months with combination therapy (P = not significant), but there was insufficient power to detect a difference.

Several retrospective analyses of randomized trials have compared survival and toxicity of combination chemoradiation between elderly and younger patients, but results have been conflicting (**Table 1**). The RTOG 94-10 trial randomly assigned patients to one of three arms: sequential chemotherapy followed by radiation therapy, concurrent chemoradiotherapy with daily radiation, or concurrent chemoradiotherapy with twice-daily radiation. A review of patients older than age 70 years enrolled in this study demonstrated increased acute toxicity, including grade 3 esophagitis and grade 3 neutropenia, in elderly patients relative to younger patients. Nonetheless, there was a survival benefit with concurrent chemoradiation therapy, with no increase in long-term toxicity, and the authors therefore conclude that combined modality therapy is a reasonable option in fit elderly patients.[27] A similar conclusion was drawn by Schild and colleagues[28] in a retrospective analysis of a phase III trial comparing concurrent chemotherapy with daily or twice-daily radiation

Table 1
Retrospective subgroup analyses of elderly patients in radiation trials for locally advanced non-small cell lung cancer

Author and Reference Number	Studies	Survival	Toxicity
Movsas et al[30]	Six phase II and III trials comparing radiation and sequential versus concurrent chemoradiation	Elderly patients over 70 years of age had best quality-adjusted survival with radiation, whereas younger patients did best with chemoradiation	Not included
Werner-Wasik et al[8]	Nine phase I–III trials involving radiation with or without chemotherapy	Better survival in young patients than in elderly patients; elderly patients with excellent performance status benefited from addition of chemotherapy	Not included
Langer, et al[2]	Three phase II–III trials comparing radiation and sequential versus concurrent chemoradiation	Elderly patients did not benefit from sequential or concurrent chemoradiation as compared with radiation alone	Significantly increased grade 4 and 5 toxicity in elderly patients receiving chemoradiation versus radiation alone
Langer, et al[27]	Phase III trial comparing sequential versus concurrent daily or twice-daily chemoradiation	Median survival 22.4 months in daily-radiation arm, 16.4 months in twice-daily radiation arm, and 10.8 months in sequential radiation arm	Increased acute toxicity in elderly patients relative to younger patients but no difference in long-term toxicity
Schild et al[28]	Phase III trial comparing daily versus twice-daily concurrent chemoradiation	Survival in elderly patients equivalent to that in younger patients	Increased toxicity, especially myelosuppression and pneumonitis in elderly patients
Rocha-Lima et al[29]	Phase III trial comparing sequential versus concurrent chemoradiation	Survival in elderly equivalent to that in younger patients	Increased grade 3+ hematologic and grade 3+ renal toxicity in elderly patients

in patients who had stage III NSCLC. Overall survival at 2 and 5 years was 39% and 18%, respectively, in patients younger than age 70 years and 36% and 13%, respectively, in patients age 70 years or older (P = not significant). Again, there was significantly greater acute toxicity in elderly patients, but, given the survival benefit, the authors conclude that combined modality therapy is appropriate in fit elderly patients.

An additional retrospective analysis was performed on the Cancer and Leukemia Group B phase III trial 9130, which randomly assigned patients who had stage III NSCLC to sequential cisplatin and vinblastine followed by radiation therapy or to concurrent cisplatin, vinblastine, and radiation therapy. The results were consistent with those reported by Langer and colleagues[27] and Schild and colleagues[28] in finding significantly increased hematologic and renal toxicity but no difference in overall survival or response rates in elderly patients compared with younger patients.[29] Werner-Wasik and colleagues[8] analyzed data from nine RTOG trials in which patients who had locally advanced NSCLC received radiation with or without chemotherapy. Chemotherapy was given either as induction therapy, concurrently with radiation, or both. Recursive partitioning analysis identified five patient subgroups with significantly different median survival times. Patients who had excellent performance status had higher median survival with the addition of chemotherapy, regardless of age (median survival of 16.2 months with chemotherapy, versus 11.9 months without chemotherapy). Patients who had Karnofsky performance status scores less than 90 and who were older than 70 years of age fell into the two subgroups with the lowest median survival times, 5.6 to 6.4 months and 2.9 months, respectively, depending on whether pleural effusion was absent or present. There was no analysis of toxicity rates in this study.

At least one study presented findings contradictory to those discussed above. Movsas and colleagues[30] retrospectively analyzed six phase II and phase III trials enrolling 979 patients who had stage II–IIIB inoperable NSCLC. They reported a significant improvement in median survival and quality-adjusted survival with combination chemoradiotherapy in patients younger than age 60 years but better quality-adjusted survival with radiation alone in patients older than age 70 years. There was a trend toward improved outcome with more aggressive therapy in patients between the ages of 60 and 70 years.

The benefit of chemoradiation therapy in elderly patients who have locally advanced NSCLC therefore remains unclear, because of the paucity of elderly-specific data and because of conflicting results within the available data. Given the available data, combined-modality therapy should be considered in fit elderly patients who have good performance status, but the toxicity of such therapy in patients who have comorbidities or poor performance status should be weighed, along with the lack of data demonstrating benefit. Randomized clinical trials designed specifically for the latter group of elderly patients will be critical in identifying the optimal therapeutic regimen.

Small Cell Lung Cancer

Limited-stage disease

Small cell lung cancer (SCLC) is classified as limited or extensive stage, depending upon whether the extent of disease can be encompassed safely in a single radiation port, generally confined to one hemithorax. The standard therapy for limited-stage SCLC involves four to six cycles of platinum-based chemotherapy with concurrent radiation therapy followed by prophylactic cranial irradiation in patients achieving a complete response to chemoradiotherapy. The benefit of thoracic radiation in limited-stage SCLC was established by a meta-analysis by Pignon and colleagues[31] that reviewed 13 randomized trials enrolling a total of 2140 patients. The relative risk of death in the group receiving chemoradiation therapy compared with the group receiving chemotherapy alone was 0.86. This risk corresponded to a 14% decrease in the mortality rate and a 3-year overall survival benefit of 5.4% ± 1.4%. The improvement, however, did not persist when considering exclusively patients over the age of 70 years.

The standard of care for limited-stage SCLC also is based on the Intergroup Trial 0096 in which patients were treated with four cycles of cisplatin and etoposide and were assigned randomly to concurrent thoracic radiation either once or twice daily to 45 Gy. Twice-daily radiation improved 5-year overall survival rates from 16% to 26% and decreased local recurrence rates from 52% to 36% ($P = .06$).[32] Yuen and colleagues[33] performed a subset analysis of this randomized trial, comparing the outcomes of the 50 patients older than 70 years with those of the 331 patients younger than 70 years. They found a significant increase in grade 4 or 5 hematologic toxicity (61% versus 84%, $P < .01$) and fatal toxicity (1% versus 10%, $P = .01$) in elderly patients. Five-year overall survival was better in younger patients (22% versus 16%, $P = .05$), but there was no difference in 5-year event-free survival, response rate, time to local failure, or duration of response.

Similar results were reported by Schild and colleagues[34] in analyzing the North Central Cancer Treatment Group protocol 89-20-52, which randomly assigned patients to daily or twice-daily thoracic radiation with concurrent cisplatin and etoposide chemotherapy. There was no difference in 5-year overall survival between patients younger or older than age 70 years (17% versus 22%, respectively, $P = .14$), but there were significantly higher rates of grade 4 or greater pneumonitis (0% versus 6%, $P = .008$) and significantly higher rates of grade 5 toxicity (0.5% versus 5.6%, $P = .03$) in patients over age 70 years.

Because of these toxicities, two small phase II trials have explored potentially less aggressive regimens to treat elderly patients who have limited-stage SCLC (**Table 2**). Jeremic and colleagues[35] treated patients with two cycles of etoposide plus carboplatin with accelerated hyperfractionated radiation (45 Gy in 1.5-Gy fractions, twice daily) and report a response rate of 75% with complete response in 57%. Two- and 5-year overall survival rates were 32% and 13%, respectively, and acute toxicity was acceptable. Murray and colleagues[36] administered one cycle of cyclophosphamide plus doxorubicin and one cycle of cisplatin plus etoposide with reduced-dose thoracic radiation (20 Gy in 5 fractions or 30 Gy in 10 fractions). They report a response rate of 89% with a 51% complete response rate. Two- and 5-year overall survival rates were 28% and 18%, respectively, and toxicity was limited. These data suggest that alternative-fractionation schedules with short-course chemotherapy provide reasonable alternatives for limiting the toxicity of standard therapy in treating elderly patients who have limited-stage SCLC.

Regardless of the fractionation schedule, there is strong evidence that patients who have a complete response to chemoradiation therapy benefit from prophylactic cranial irradiation (PCI). Auperin and colleagues[37] conducted a meta-analysis of seven trials that randomly assigned patients who had limited-stage SCLC and a complete response to chemoradiation therapy to PCI or to no PCI. They report a 5.4% increase in 3-year overall survival with PCI, which was not affected by age. At the same time, clinical trials have demonstrated short-term memory deficits and long-term neuropsychologic deficits as a result of cranial radiation.[38] Because the elderly population is at increased risk of baseline cognitive impairment, proper selection criteria are needed to determine which elderly patients are appropriate candidates for PCI.

Palliative Radiation Therapy

In extensive-stage SCLC and metastatic NSCLC, thoracic radiation is used for palliation of symptoms such as cough, hemoptysis, chest pain, dyspnea, or airway obstruction. Randomized, controlled trials evaluating various fractionation regimens for palliation of symptoms have had conflicting results,[39] but there is some evidence that high-dose radiation may be associated with improved survival over lower-dose radiation.[40–42] A meta-analysis performed by Fairchild and colleagues[39] reported equivalence of palliation of specific symptoms with high-dose and low-dose radiation but a lower total symptom score after high-dose palliative radiation. Furthermore, they found a 4.8% increase in 1-year overall survival

Table 2
Phase II chemoradiation trials in elderly patients who had limited-stage small cell lung cancer

Study	Number of Patients	Age (Years)	Chemotherapy	Radiation Dose (Gy)	Percent Objective Response (Complete + Partial)	Median Survival (Months)	5-year Overall Survival Rate (%)
Murray et al[36]	55	>70	Cyclophosphamide, doxorubicin, vincristine × one cycle + etoposide, cisplatin × one cycle	20–30	89 (51 + 38)	12.6	18
Jeremic et al[35]	72	>70	Etoposide, cisplatin × one cycle	45 accelerated hyper-fractionation	75 (57 + 18)	15	13

with fractionation schedules of 35 Gy_{10} biologically equivalent dose. There was, however, increased esophagitis with the high-dose regimens.

Turner and colleagues[43] performed a prospective observational cohort study of patients receiving palliative thoracic radiation, comparing the response to treatment and European Organization for the Research and Treatment of Cancer quality-of-life scores for patients younger than age 65 years and patients older than age 75 years. They found no significant difference in toxicity between the two arms. They conclude that elderly patients should be treated with the same palliative regimens as younger patients and should be expected to experience a similar benefit.

In conclusion, available data regarding the appropriateness of standard radiation therapy approaches in the treatment of elderly patients are conflicting. Results are consistent, however, in demonstrating increased toxicity in this patient population, probably as a result decreased baseline performance status and increased medical comorbidities. The remainder of this article therefore reviews toxicity associated with thoracic irradiation and methods that have been developed to limit these effects.

TOXICITY OF THORACIC IRRADIATION

As discussed in the previous sections, thoracic irradiation is a mainstay of therapy for lung cancer. Its use, however, is frequently limited by concern for toxicity. Radiation-induced lung injury is particularly important in elderly patients, because they often present with medical comorbidities and compromised baseline pulmonary function. This section reviews the presentation and mechanism of the dose-limiting toxicities associated with thoracic irradiation.

Pulmonary Toxicity

Pulmonary toxicity associated with thoracic irradiation is generally classified as either acute or late. Clinically, acute radiation pneumonitis after fractionated therapy is associated with fever, nonproductive cough, and dyspnea within several months after completion of radiation. It typically resolves without sequelae within 6 to 8 weeks. Histologically, this syndrome is believed to be a bilateral lymphocytic alveolitis or hypersensitivity pneumonitis, involving both irradiated and non-irradiated segments of the lung.[44–46] Classical pneumonitis is associated with volume of lung irradiated and threshold dose and has a sigmoid dose–response curve with rapidly rising morbidity leading to death over a small dose range.[44,47] This type of pneumonitis is associated with initial damage to pneumocytes and endothelial cells with surfactant release into alveoli, followed by an inflammatory response with an influx of leukocytes, plasma cells, macrophages, fibroblasts, and collagen fibers. The end result is fibrosis with loss of capillaries, thickening of the alveolar septa, and narrowing of the alveolar space.[44]

Late radiation toxicity is manifested most commonly as pulmonary fibrosis. It is a result of repair of tissue injury and varies with the severity and frequency of the injury. The mechanism seems to involve a cytokine cascade including transforming growth factor beta, leading to fibroblast synthesis of collagen.[48] Unlike pneumonitis, pulmonary fibrosis is found only in irradiated areas of the lung. Clinically, it presents with a gradual and persistent onset of shortness of breath, with the majority of symptomatic patients presenting within 6 months of completion of therapy. Objectively, late pulmonary fibrosis is associated with a decrease in the transfer factor (DLCO) with relatively little change in the forced expiratory volume in 1 second on pulmonary function tests.[49] A statistically significant correlation has been found between the reduction in DLCO and the volume of lung receiving more than 30 Gy (V30) on the dose–volume histogram in patients who had a pre-radiation DLCO greater than 50% of the predicted value.[50] A multivariate analysis of patients receiving chemotherapy in conjunction with radiation therapy also suggested that fractions greater than 2.67 Gy are associated with an increased risk of late pulmonary fibrosis.[51]

In general, late pulmonary fibrosis is the dose-limiting toxicity in radiation for lung tumors. This experience suggests that dose per fraction and lung V30 are the most important factors in evaluating the safety of a plan in an elderly patient who has compromised baseline pulmonary function.

Non-Pulmonary Toxicity

Esophagitis is another dose-limiting toxicity associated with thoracic irradiation. It can cause dehydration and weight loss necessitating treatment interruptions. Elderly patients have higher rates of frailty and malnourishment at baseline than younger patients, and as a result esophagitis may be particularly problematic. If poor oral caloric intake is a concern, consideration should be given to placement of a prophylactic feeding tube for nutritional supplementation. Maintenance intravenous fluid administration may also be required.

Radiation-associated toxicity generally is the result of radiation dose and the volume of normal tissue irradiated. Therefore, the dose-limiting toxicities discussed previously, such as pneumonitis, pulmonary fibrosis, and esophagitis, can be reduced or avoided by limiting radiation exposure. This discussion next explores methods designed to decrease radiation to organs adjacent to tumors, thereby limiting toxicity and allowing improved safety and efficacy of radiation therapy in elderly patients.

TECHNICAL ADVANCES IN RADIATION THERAPY

Technical advances in radiation oncology allow the reduction in normal tissue toxicity in treatment of thoracic tumors. Because increased toxicity is a particular concern in elderly patients, these methods may be particularly important in increasing the tolerability of therapy in these patients.

Radiation treatment plans typically include the gross tumor with extra margin around the tumor to account for uncertainties such as tumor motion with respiration, microscopic spread of disease, and daily set-up error in positioning the patient. This volume, known as the "planning target volume" (PTV), is always larger than the extent of disease seen on imaging studies and leads to increased radiation dose to normal structures and increased normal tissue toxicity. Methods of decreasing the PTV include minimizing tumor movement, increasing set-up accuracy, and maximizing dose conformity with rapid dose falloff.

Over the past few years, four-dimensional respiration-correlated CT (4D-CT) has become used increasingly to observe and quantify tumor motion. With this technology, the respiratory waveform is recorded for a minimum of one full respiratory cycle, and the images are sorted into conventional three-dimensional CT scans representative of the patient's anatomy at each of 10 phases of the respiratory cycle. This imaging allows reduction of the treatment margin to correspond with the true extent of tumor motion. 4D-CT scans also are used to stratify radiation treatment approaches by determining which patients have large respiratory-induced motion and therefore would benefit from strategies such as active breathing control, diaphragm control, or respiratory gating. All these techniques minimize organ motion, thereby allowing a reduction in the PTV and a decrease in the volume of irradiated normal tissue.

A second method of reducing the PTV is by improving set-up accuracy. One way of increasing accuracy is with image-guided radiation therapy, which uses kilovoltage or megavoltage imaging devices integrated into the linear accelerator to allow close monitoring of patient and tumor position, permitting a reduction in the safety margin. Another emerging technology is adaptive radiation therapy in which the treatment plan is modified to account for changes such as growth or shrinkage of the tumor, increase or decrease in atelectasis, or excessive weight loss, again allowing smaller initial planning margins.[52]

Limiting the volume of normal tissues exposed to radiation through the aforementioned techniques allows hypofractionation to be employed. The use of hypofractionation has a theoretical benefit in tumor control by decreasing accelerated repopulation of tumor cells and minimizing repair of radiation-induced damage to tumor cells, thereby achieving exponential cell killing. Hypofractionation shortens the overall treatment time and is more convenient for patients, a consideration that may be of increased importance in the elderly, for whom mobility often is more difficult and transportation challenges are more common.

Data regarding the efficacy and toxicity of stereotactic body radiotherapy (SBRT) are promising. Brock and colleagues[53] conducted a review of published studies on hypofractionated SBRT in patients who had localized NSCLC and report a weighted 2-year survival rate of 65% and a 2-year local progression-free survival rate of 89%. The incidence of grade 2 or greater symptomatic pneumonitis ranged from 0 to 29%, with a weighted mean of 6.5%. Esophagitis was transient, and late toxicities were rare. Catastrophic toxicity was reported in only one study in which a patient died of a bleeding esophageal ulcer after receiving 48 Gy in eight fractions for a central tumor. These data are promising and suggest that SBRT may be a reasonable method to improve convenience and toxicity associated with radiation therapy, without significantly compromising tumor control. Trials comparing hypofractionated radiation with standard fractionation schedules will be critical in confirming these results, and elderly-specific trials would be useful to confirm that the results are applicable to older patients.

In conclusion, radiation-associated toxicity may be limited by using a variety of techniques including respiration-correlated 4D-CT scanning, image guidance, adaptive radiotherapy, and SBRT, all of which can be used to limit the radiation dose received by normal structures. Decreased irradiation of organs adjacent to the tumor may allow hypofractionation, which has an added benefit of increased convenience. Because of the increased concern about radiation-induced toxicity in elderly patients, these technologies play a critical role in improving the feasibility of radiation therapy in this patient population.

SUMMARY

This article has reviewed radiation treatment of thoracic malignancies in elderly patients. In general the literature suggests that thoracic irradiation is equally efficacious in elderly patients as in younger patients and is associated with increased but acceptable toxicity. Technical advances are allowing a further reduction in morbidity with preliminary results suggestive of stable outcomes. Prospective data from elderly specific trials are needed to determine the optimal treatment of lung cancer and to compare innovative radiation technology with standard therapies.

REFERENCES

1. Havlik RJ, Yancik R, Long S, et al. The National Cancer Institute on Aging and the National Cancer Institute SEER collaborative study on comorbidity and early diagnosis of cancer in the elderly. Cancer 1994;74(Suppl 7):2101–6.
2. Langer C, Scott C, Byhardt R. Effect of advanced age on outcome in Radiation Therapy Oncology Group studies of locally advanced NSCLC. Lung Cancer 2000;29(Suppl 1):119.
3. Ries LAG, Eisner MP, Kosary CL, et al. SEER cancer statistics review 1975–2000. Available at: http://seer.cancer.gov/csr/1975_2000. Accessed October 28, 2008.
4. Wingo PA, Cardinez CJ, Landis SH, et al. Long term trends in cancer mortality in the United States, 1930–1998. Cancer 2003;97(Suppl 12):3133–275.
5. Zeber JE, Copeland LA, Hosek BJ, et al. Cancer rates, medical comorbidities, and treatment modalities in the oldest patients. Crit Rev Oncol Hematol 2008;67:237–42.
6. Paesmans M, Sculier JP, Libert G, et al. Prognostic factors for survival in advanced non-small-cell lung cancer: univariate and multivariate analyses including recursive partitioning and amalgamation algorithms in 1,052 patients. J Clin Oncol 1995;13:1221–30.
7. Albain KS, Crowley JJ, LeBlanc M, et al. Survival determinants in extensive-stage non–small-cell lung cancer: the Southwest Oncology Group experience. Am J Clin Oncol 1991;9:1618–26.
8. Werner-Wasik M, Scott C, Cox JD, et al. Recursive partitioning analysis of 1999 Radiation Therapy Oncology Group (RTOG) patients with locally-advanced non-small-cell lung cancer (LA-NSCLC): identification of five groups with different survival. Int J Radiat Oncol Biol Phys 2000;48(5):1475–82.
9. Jatoi A, Hillman S, Stella P, et al. Should elderly non-small-cell lung cancer patients be offered elderly-specific trials? Results of a pooled analysis from the North Central Cancer Treatment Group. J Clin Oncol 2005;23(36):9113–9.
10. Cheung PC, Makillop WJ, Dixon P, et al. Involved-field radiotherapy alone for early-stage non-small-cell lung cancer. Int J Radiat Oncol Biol Phys 2000;48(3):703–10.
11. Hayakawa K, Mitsuhashi N, Saito Y, et al. Limited field irradiation for medically inoperable patients with peripheral stage I non-small cell lung cancer. Lung Cancer 1999;26(3):137–42.
12. Krol AD, Aussems P, Noordijk EM, et al. Local irradiation alone for peripheral stage I lung cancer: could we omit the elective regional nodal irradiation? Int J Radiat Oncol Biol Phys 1996;34(2):297–302.
13. Noordijk EM, vd Poest Clement E, Hermans J, et al. Radiotherapy as an alternative to surgery in elderly patients with resectable lung cancer. Radiother Oncol 1988;13(2):83–9.
14. Hayakawa K, Mitsuhashi N, Katano S, et al. High-dose radiation therapy for elderly patients with inoperable or unresectable non-small cell lung cancer. Lung Cancer 2001;32:81–8.
15. Gauden SJ, Tripcony L. The curative treatment by radiation therapy alone of stage I non-small cell lung cancer in a geriatric population. Lung Cancer 2001;32:71–9.
16. Yu HM, Liu YF, Yu JM, et al. Involved-field radiotherapy is effective for patients 70 years old or more with early stage non-small cell lung cancer. Radiother Oncol 2008;87:29–34.
17. Furuse K, Fukuoka M, Kawahara M, et al. Phase III study of concurrent versus sequential thoracic radiotherapy in combination with mitomycin, vindesine, and cisplatin in unresectable stage III non-small-cell lung cancer. J Clin Oncol 1999;17(9):2692–9.
18. Curran W, Scott C, Langer C. Long-term benefit is observed in phase III comparison of sequential versus concurrent chemo-radiation for patients with unresected stage III NSCLC: RTOG 9410. [abstract]. Proc Am Soc Clin Oncol 2003;22:621.
19. Fournel P, Robinet G, Thomas P, et al. Randomized phase III trial of sequential chemoradiotherapy compared with concurrent chemoradiotherapy in locally advanced non-small-cell lung cancer: Groupe Français de Pneumo-Cancerlolgie NPC 95-01 Study. J Clin Oncol 2005;23(25):5910–7.
20. Zatloukal P, Petruzelka L, Zemanova M, et al. Concurrent versus sequential chemoradiotherapy with cisplatin and vinorelbine in locally advanced non-small cell lung cancer: a randomized study. Lung Cancer 2004;46(1):97–8.
21. Semrau S, Klautke G, Virchow JC, et al. Impact of comorbidity and age on the outcome of patients with inoperable NSCLC treated with concurrent chemoradiotherapy. Respir Med 2008;102:210–8.
22. Semrau S, Bier A, Thierbach U, et al. Concurrent radiochemotherapy with vinorelbine plus cisplatin or carboplatin in patients with locally advanced non-small-cell lung cancer (NSCLC) and increased risk

of treatment complications. Preliminary results. Strahlenther Onkol 2003;179(12):823–31.

23. Lau DH, Crowley JJ, Gandara DR, et al. Southwest Oncology Group phase II trial of concurrent carboplatin, etoposide, and radiation for poor-risk stage III non-small-cell lung cancer. J Clin Oncol 1998; 16(9):3078–81.
24. Cardenel F, Arnaiz MD, Isla D. Randomized phase II study of sequential versus concurrent chemoradiotherapy in poor-risk patients with inoperable stage III non-small cell lung cancer [abstract]. Proc Am Soc Clin Oncol 2005;24:7255.
25. Semrau S, Bier A, Thierbach U, et al. 6-Year experience of concurrent radiochemotherapy with vinorelbine plus a platinum compound in multimorbid or aged patients with inoperable non-small cell lung cancer. Strahlenther Onkol 2007;183(1):30–5.
26. Atagi S, Kawahara M, Ogawara M, et al. Standard thoracic radiotherapy with or without concurrent daily low-dose carboplatin in elderly patients with locally advanced non-small cell lung cancer: a phase III trial of the Japan Clinical Oncology Group (JCOG9812). Jpn J Clin Oncol 2005;35:195–201.
27. Langer CJ, Hsu C, Curran WJ. Elderly patients with locally advanced non-small cell lung cancer benefit from combined modality therapy: secondary analysis of Radiation Therapy Oncology Group (RTOG) 94-10 [abstract]. Proc Am Soc Clin Oncol 2002; 21(299a):1193.
28. Schild SE, Stella PJ, Geyer SM, et al. The outcome of combined-modality therapy for stage III non-small-cell lung cancer in the elderly. J Clin Oncol 2003; 21(17):3201–6.
29. Rocha Lima CM, Herndon JE II, Kosty M, et al. Therapy choices among older patients with lung carcinoma: an evaluation of two trials of the Cancer and Leukemia Group B. Cancer 2002;94(1):181–7.
30. Movsas B, Scott C, Sause W, et al. The benefit of treatment intensification is age and histology-dependent in patients with locally advanced non-small cell lung cancer (NSCLC): a quality-adjusted survival analysis of Radiation Therapy Oncology Group (RTOG) chemoradiation studies. Int J Radiat Oncol Biol Phys 1999;45(5):1143–9.
31. Pignon JP, Arriagada R, Ihde DC, et al. A meta-analysis of thoracic radiotherapy for small-cell lung cancer. N Engl J Med 1992;327(23):1618–24.
32. Turrisi AT, Kim K, Blum R, et al. Twice-daily compared with once-daily thoracic radiotherapy in limited small-cell lung cancer treated concurrently with cisplatin and etoposide. N Engl J Med 1999; 340:265–71.
33. Yuen AR, Zou G, Turrisi AT, et al. Similar outcome of elderly patients in intergroup trial 0096: cisplatin, etoposide, and thoracic radiotherapy administered once or twice daily in limited stage small cell lung carcinoma. Cancer 2000;89(9):1953–60.
34. Schild SE, Stella PJ, Brooks BJ, et al. Results of combined-modality therapy for limited stage small cell lung carcinoma in the elderly. Cancer 2005; 103:2349–54.
35. Jeremic B, Shibamoto Y, Acimovic L, et al. Carboplatin, etoposide, and accelerated hyperfractionated radiotherapy for elderly patients with limited small cell lung carcinoma: a phase II study. Cancer 1998;82(5):836–41.
36. Murray N, Grafton C, Shah A, et al. Abbreviated treatment for elderly, infirm, or noncompliant patients with limited stage small cell lung cancer. J Clin Oncol 1998;16(10):3323–8.
37. Auperin A, Arriagada R, Pignon JP, et al. Prophylactic cranial irradiation for patients with small cell lung cancer in complete remission. Prophylactic Cranial Irradiation Overview Collaborative Group. N Engl J Med 1999;341:476–84.
38. Crossen JR, Garwood D, Glastien E, et al. Neurobehavioral sequelae of cranial irradiation in adults: a review of radiation induced encephalopathy. J Clin Oncol 1994;12(3):627–42.
39. Fairchild A, Harris K, Barnes E, et al. Palliative thoracic radiotherapy for lung cancer: a systematic review. J Clin Oncol 2008;26(24):4001–11.
40. Medical Research Council Lung Cancer Working Party. Randomized trial of palliative two-fraction versus more intensive 13-fraction radiotherapy for patients with inoperable non-small cell lung cancer and good performance status. Clin Oncol 1996;8: 167–75.
41. Bezjak A, Dixon P, Brundage M, et al. Randomized phase III trial of single versus fractionated thoracic radiation in the palliation of patients with lung cancer. Int J Radiat Oncol Biol Phys 2002;54(3):719–28.
42. Kramer GW, Wanders SL, Noordijk EM, et al. Results of the Dutch National study of the palliative effect of irradiation using two different treatment schemes for non-small cell lung cancer. J Clin Oncol 2005; 23(13):2962–70.
43. Turner NJ, Muers MF, Haward RA, et al. Do elderly people with lung cancer benefit from palliative radiotherapy? Lung Cancer 2005;49:193–202.
44. Abratt RP, Morgan GW. Lung toxicity following chest irradiation in patients with lung cancer. Lung Cancer 2002;35:103–9.
45. Gibson PG, Bryant DH, Morgan GW, et al. Radiation-induced lung injury: a hypersensitivity pneumonitis? Ann Intern Med 1988;109:288–91.
46. Nakayama Y, Makino S, Fukuda Y, et al. Activation of lavage lymphocytes in lung injuries caused by radiotherapy for lung cancer. Int J Radiat Oncol Biol Phys 1996;34:459–67.
47. Travis EL, Tucker SL. The relationship between functional assays of radiation response in the lung and target cell depletion. Br J Cancer 1986;53(Suppl 7):304–19.

48. Rubin P, Johnston CJ, Williams JP, et al. A perpetual cascade of cytokines post-irradiation leads to pulmonary fibrosis. Int J Radiat Oncol Biol Phys 1995;33:99–109.
49. Abratt RP, Wilcox PA. The effect of irradiation on lung function and perfusion in patients with lung cancer. Int J Radiat Oncol Biol Phys 1995;31:915–9.
50. Kwa SLS, Lebesque JV, Theuws JCM, et al. Radiation pneumonitis as a function of mean lung dose: an analysis of pooled data for 540 patients. Int J Radiat Oncol Biol Phys 1998;42:1–9.
51. Bria WF, Kanarek DJ, Kazemi H. Prediction of postoperative pulmonary function following thoracic operations. Value of ventilation-perfusion scanning. J Thorac Cardiovasc Surg 1983;86:186–92.
52. Fox J, Ford E, Redmond K, et al. Quantification of lung tumor volume changes during radiotherapy for non-small cell lung cancer. Int J Radiat Oncol Biol Phys 2009;74(2):341–8.
53. Brock J, Ashley S, Bedford J, et al. Review of hypofractionated small volume radiotherapy for early-stage non-small cell lung cancer. Clin Oncol 2008; doi:10.1016/j.clon.2008.06.005. Accessed June 8, 2009.

Quality of Life and Ethical Concerns in the Elderly Thoracic Surgery Patient

Holly M. Holmes, MD

KEYWORDS

- Elderly • Quality of life • Pulmonary surgery
- Life expectancy • Geriatric assessment

The burden of lung disease is high in the elderly. More than half of lung cancers are diagnosed in patients older than 65 years,[1] and older persons have a high prevalence of chronic obstructive pulmonary disease.[2] As the population ages, treatment of lung diseases must focus increasingly on how to risk-stratify older patients for particular therapies and how to ensure that age-specific outcomes are measured and achieved.[3] Older patients have higher complication rates, lower long-term survival rates, and more comorbidity than younger patients.[1] Thus, a consideration of how to provide the best treatment for an older patient must take into account the unique challenges presented by the aging population.

THE ELDERLY POPULATION IS INCREASING RAPIDLY

In the United States, more than 80 million people will be 65 years and older by 2050.[4] Providing optimal therapy to the elderly requires recognition that elderly persons are not merely older adults. Because of the burdens of comorbidity, age-related physiologic changes, differences in functional status, and geriatric-specific conditions, the elderly population is a heterogeneous group.[5] Incorporating a comprehensive geriatric assessment into the evaluation of every elderly patient considered a candidate for thoracic surgery may be logistically difficult and may be an overuse of valuable resources.[6] Because there are only 3.9 geriatricians for every 10,000 persons 75 years and older in the United States,[7] incorporating a geriatrics consultation into every thoracic surgery patient's care is equally unrealistic. Therefore, increasingly, the challenge will be to "geriatricize" medical and surgical disciplines to incorporate targeted assessments and specialized care of the elderly into treatment trials and clinical practice.

LONG-TERM SURVIVAL IN LUNG CANCER REMAINS LOW

Between 2001 and 2005, the median age at diagnosis of lung cancer was 71 years, and the median age at death was 72 years.[8] Despite significant improvement in long-term survival for many common cancers in the elderly, survival for patients who have lung cancer remains low.[9] The 5-year survival rate for patients after surgery for early-stage lung cancer in the Surveillance Epidemiology and End Results[8] (SEER) Program was 65.2% in persons younger than 67 years and 51.5% for those 67 years and older.[10] Survival was associated with tumor size, gender, age, and the extent of the resection.[10] Older patients may be offered less extensive resections because of high operative risk or comorbidity.[10] **Fig. 1** shows the trends in overall 5-year survival for patients who have lung cancer by age in the SEER Program between 1975 and 2000.[11]

Holly M. Holmes is supported by a Hartford Geriatrics Health Outcomes Research Scholars Award.
Department of General Internal Medicine, Ambulatory Treatment and Emergency Care, The University of Texas M. D. Anderson Cancer Center, 1515 Holcombe Boulevard, Unit 1465, Houston, TX 77030, USA
E-mail address: hholmes@mdanderson.org

Thorac Surg Clin 19 (2009) 401–407
doi:10.1016/j.thorsurg.2009.06.001

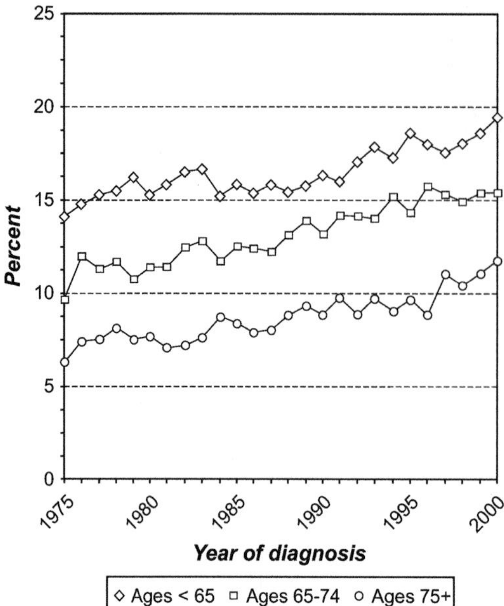

Fig. 1. Trends in 5-year survival for patients who had lung cancer by age at diagnosis from 1975 to 2000 according to SEER. Despite an overall increase in 5-year survival, survival rates are lower in patients aged 65 to 74 years and older than 75 years than in younger patients. (*Adapted from* The Surveillance Epidemiology and End Results Program, Available at: http://seer.cancer.gov/faststats/. Accessed February 2009.)

AGE ALONE IS NOT A CONTRAINDICATION TO THORACIC SURGERY IN THE ELDERLY

Several studies have demonstrated that age alone should not exclude a patient from lung surgery.[12–14] Older patients who undergo resection for lung cancer have reasonable short- and long-term morbidity and mortality rates when compared with younger patients.[15–17] Predictors of operative mortality include tumor stage, performance status, and weight loss.[18] Perioperative and early postoperative mortality range from 2.6% to 9.5%.[19,20] Emergency surgery, comorbidity (including cardiac disease), more advanced cancer stage, and extent of resection are associated with early postoperative mortality.[19,21–24] Neoadjuvant chemotherapy also was associated with postoperative morbidity in a study of 726 patients undergoing resection for non-small cell lung cancer, about half of whom were age 70 years or older.[17] Existing data on surgery in the elderly support the conclusion that cancer stage and comorbidities are more important than age alone in predicting long-term survival,[19,21] and extent of resection is important in predicting perioperative morbidity and mortality. Hence, elderly patients are excluded from surgery on the basis of performance status and comorbidity rather than age alone.[25]

THE ROLE OF QUALITY-OF-LIFE ASSESSMENT IN THORACIC SURGERY

Patients who have lung cancer or chronic obstructive lung disease typically have a lower baseline quality of life (QOL) than their peers.[26–28] Age and comorbidities impair QOL as measured by the Short Form-36, a general QOL scale.[9] Symptom burden is especially high in patients who have lung cancer, and dyspnea, which correlates with poor QOL, is a common symptom for older persons diagnosed with lung cancer.[3,9] Patients who have lung cancer may have an impaired QOL because of lower levels of physical function, low emotional role functioning, impaired mental health, and low energy compared with the population.[28] They also may have other smoking-related comorbidities, such as coronary artery disease and peripheral arterial disease, as well as a high incidence of other cancers, all of which diminish QOL.[3] In a study of 112 patients who had lung cancer, QOL was impaired compared with the population in seven of eight subscales (the exception was the subscale for pain). This study, however, measured QOL once at a mean of 23 months after thoracic surgery.[27] Lung cancer survivors have more physical and psychosocial problems than survivors of prostate and colon cancer.[9]

Although resection of a lung tumor may provide the best chance for substantial survival, the potential detriment to QOL in patients undergoing thoracic surgery has been a concern, because these patients already have a markedly diminished QOL.[9] Most studies of QOL in thoracic surgery have focused on QOL before and months after resection for lung cancer. Several general and cancer-specific scales to measure QOL are summarized in **Table 1**.

THE EFFECT OF THORACIC SURGERY ON QOL

Quality of life decreases after thoracic surgery and generally returns to baseline over a period of 3 to 9 months after surgery.[37] Although different general and disease-specific scales have been used to measure QOL, most studies of QOL after thoracic surgery have shown a decrease from baseline QOL over the first 3 months after surgery. This decline lasts approximately 3 months and returns to baseline within 9 months after surgery.[38] Poor QOL after surgery has been associated with symptoms of dyspnea, depression, nausea, and pain and has been correlated with larger resections[38] but not necessarily with pulmonary function. One study demonstrating a decline in physical and social functioning, mental health, and pain scores at 6 months postoperatively showed no association

Table 1
Common assessment tools for measuring quality of life

Instrument	Description	Target Population
European Organization for Research and Treatment of Cancer Quality of Life Questionnaire-C30 (EORTC QLQ-C30)[29]	30 questions covering physical, social, emotional functioning, and global quality of life	Patients who have cancer
European Organization for Research and Treatment of Cancer Quality of Life Questionnaire-LC13[30]	13-item measure of lung cancer–specific symptoms, meant to be used in conjunction with the EORTC QLQ-C30	Patients who have lung cancer
Functional Assessment of Cancer Therapy–Lung (FACT-L) Questionnaire[31]	34 questions with five subscales, including physical, social, emotional, and functional well-being, as well as a lung cancer subscale	Patients who have lung cancer
Functional Living Index – Cancer (FLI-C)[32]	22 questions, divided into physical well-being and ability factors and emotional state factors	Patients who have cancer
Lung Cancer Symptom Scale (LCSS)[33]	9 items measuring symptoms, activity level, and overall quality of life	Patients who have lung cancer
Short Form 36 (SF-36)[34]	36 questions and eight scales, including physical and mental health	General
Short Form 36 version 2 (SF-36v2)[35]	SF-36 divided into physical and mental health component scales that can be independently weighted and compared	General
Sickness Impact Profile (SIP)[36]	136 items in 12 categories, including self-assessment of sickness and dysfunction, physical dimensions, and independent categories	General

with measures of pulmonary function.[28] In another study of 191 patients who had non-small cell lung cancer, physical function declined 1 month postoperatively but recovered at 3 months, and mental health was not diminished. Pneumonectomy was associated with lower physical function.[20]

THE EFFECT OF THORACIC SURGERY ON QOL IN THE ELDERLY

QOL has been evaluated in few trials of lung surgery in the elderly.[39] The effect of thoracic surgery on QOL does not seem to differ between older and younger patients undergoing thoracic surgery; however, studies generally have not been designed to test differences in QOL between older and younger groups.[39] In a study of QOL in 218 patients, 85 of whom were older than 70 years of age, preoperative and 3-month postoperative composite physical and mental function scores were not different in older and younger patients.[39] In 191 patients evaluated before and 3 months after surgery, measures of physical function showed an initial decrement followed by recovery, with no difference in physical or mental subscale scores between patients more than 70 years old and younger patients.[20]

QOL AS A PREDICTOR OF SURVIVAL

Preoperative or pre-cancer diagnosis QOL also may be a predictor of survival.[40] In a study of 129 patients who had lung cancer, the preoperative QOL of 90 patients alive at 3 months after surgery was compared with that of 33 patients deceased at 3 months. Prediagnosis QOL was a predictor of survival as measured by a cancer-specific scale, but lung cancer–specific measures and performance status were not robust predictors of outcome.[41] These findings need further study before widespread QOL assessment is incorporated into the preoperative risk stratification of elderly patients.

DEPRESSION AS A COMORBIDITY DISTINCT FROM IMPAIRED QOL

The prevalence of depression in patients who have cancer is twice that in the general population, and 16% to 29% of patients who have lung cancer have depression.[42] Depression or mental health often is incorporated into measures of QOL but is not routinely diagnosed and treated in trials of thoracic surgery in the elderly. Depression has been associated with increased morbidity and mortality in other surgical patients[43,44] and in elderly patients who had breast cancer,[45] but other studies of patients receiving chemotherapy did not show depression to be an independent predictor of survival.[6] Studies of depression in patients who had lung cancer have yielded mixed results. Two studies have shown a correlation between depression and survival. Studies that did not show a correlation had groups of mixed cancer stages and used less rigorous tools to diagnose depression.[42] In a study of 94 patients with a mean age of 63.3 years, depression as measured by the Center for Epidemiology Studies–Depression Scale (CES-D) improved over a 4-month period postoperatively.[37]

QUALITY OF LIFE IN THE ELDERLY: SUMMARY

Given the available data on QOL after lung cancer resection, a reasonable hypothesis is that QOL in the groups of elderly patients currently offered thoracic surgery is not affected by patient age. Older patients have the same baseline impairment in QOL, a similar decrement after thoracic surgery, and a similar return to prior baseline levels.[20,39] Current studies of surgical outcomes and QOL measures, however, incorporate the selection of fit elderly to undergo surgery. If older patients with a higher burden of comorbid illness and functional dependence are increasingly offered surgical options, QOL will need to be evaluated using disease- and age-specific measures. To understand the effect of surgery on QOL in the elderly, the QOL in fit elderly surgical patients should be compared with the QOL in patients who are deemed unfit for surgery.[46,47]

CURRENT STUDIES OF QOL MAY NOT MATCH PATIENT PREFERENCES

Although existing QOL results might be considered reassuring, patients are not concerned about immediate or short-term operative risk. Patients are willing to accept some amount of operative risk in the treatment of life-threatening illness, especially when surgery provides the best chance for a higher survival rate in an ultimately terminal illness.[48] Patients are more interested in longer-term outcomes such as functional independence and nursing home placement.[20] Few studies have evaluated QOL for longer durations. One study evaluated QOL up to 24 months after operation in 159 patients with a mean age 63 years, most of whom had early-stage non-small cell lung cancer.[49] In contrast to other studies of shorter duration, QOL did not recover completely to perioperative levels over 24 months and was significantly worse in patients who underwent pneumonectomy rather than bilobectomy or lobectomy.

ETHICAL ISSUES IN SELECTING APPROPRIATE ELDERLY PATIENTS FOR SURGERY

Because operative outcomes data and QOL seem reasonably comparable in older and younger subjects, the conclusions to date are that the results in carefully selected, fit older patients who have early-stage disease are similar to those in younger patients. Nevertheless, diminished QOL and excess symptom burden, although possibly returning to preoperative values, still remain.[37] As minimally invasive and muscle-sparing techniques are advocated for older patients, it will become increasing important to establish the appropriate selection criteria upon which to offer surgery.[47] In planning surgery for an elderly person, one should establish whether the surgery will offer the patient a reasonable expected survival time, an acceptable risk of postoperative mortality, and preserved postoperative QOL.[50] Increasingly, surgery may be performed on elderly candidates who previously would not have been offered surgery because of comorbidities or performance status.[51]

LIMITED RESECTION: A REASONABLE TRADE-OFF IN SOME PATIENTS

Minimally invasive techniques and video-assisted thorascopic surgery (VATS) may provide older patients who traditionally would be excluded from lung surgery the opportunity for more aggressive treatment of early-stage lung cancers.[52] In one series of VATS, there was no relationship between age and morbidity and mortality, with a mortality rate of less than 1% and complication rate of 15%.[53] Limited resections may be a viable option for patients who have small tumors and for patients who otherwise would be unfit for more extensive resections; survival rates for older persons who can undergo a resection safely are similar to those for younger patients.[24]

The availability of even lower-risk techniques means that frailer candidates might be considered for surgery. This option raises the issue of when surgery will no longer benefit an older person, even in the absence of increased risk. The survival benefit of resection with lobectomy versus a more limited resection becomes significant 3 years after surgery.[47] Thus, for very elderly patients who have other comorbid illness or functional impairment and who have a diminished life expectancy even in the absence of lung cancer, a limited resection may be a viable alternative as long as the patient's life expectancy with surgery greatly exceeds that without surgery.[47]

INCORPORATING LIFE EXPECTANCY INTO THE DECISION TO PROVIDE SURGERY IN THE ELDERLY

If limited resections are to become more common, more systematic means are needed to understand remaining life expectancy. It may be surprising to learn that the average 85-year-old man will live at least 4.7 years; however, 25% of 85-year-old men will live only 2.2 years.[54] These data are based on life-expectancy tables for the general United States population. Clearly, a diagnosis of lung cancer, especially later-stage cancer, places an older person in the lowest survival quartile. A recent study exploring risk factors for mortality in the elderly uses a scoring system based on gender, age, comorbid illness, and loss of activities of daily living. The risk factors were validated in frail community-dwelling elderly and not specifically in a population with cancer. Based on this scoring system, the median survival for men 75 years and older who have cancer or chronic obstructive pulmonary disease, even without including the risk from other comorbidities and functional loss, is less than 2.5 years.[55]

AGE-SPECIFIC PREOPERATIVE ASSESSMENTS BEFORE THORACIC SURGERY

Assuming a reasonable life expectancy to warrant surgery, how should an older patient be selected to provide the longest functional life expectancy with acceptable QOL? Certainly, older patients should undergo routine preoperative assessment of pulmonary and cardiac function to determine their fitness for surgery.[56] In addition, special attention must be given to other comorbidities and functional status. Comorbidities are important determinants of surgical outcome.[25,57] In addition to QOL measured using disease-specific tools, fitness for surgery should be considered using a geriatric-specific evaluation.[6] In addition to comorbidity, geriatric conditions such as dementia, poor nutrition, impaired vision, hearing loss, dizziness, falls, and incontinence are as prevalent as common comorbidities such as heart disease or diabetes and are associated with disability,[58] but their prevalence and importance in elderly patients undergoing thoracic surgical procedures is unknown.

SUMMARY

The diversity of older patients presents a challenge when deciding whether to recommend thoracic surgery to an individual. Comparable postoperative morbidity and mortality between younger and older patient groups indicate that surgeons are skilled in determining which older patients are most fit for surgery on the basis of comorbidities, performance status, and QOL. Criteria for the inclusion of older patients in thoracic surgical trials have not been described, however. As newer, minimally invasive techniques and limited resections are incorporated into elderly patients' care, criteria for inclusion must be evaluated prospectively in trials designed to establish risk factors for morbidity and mortality in elderly patients traditionally excluded from surgery. In addition, QOL needs to be evaluated specifically in the elderly, and meaningful comparisons need to be made with other elderly patients who do not undergo surgery. Finally, to inform better the ethical debate about whether thoracic surgery benefits a patient of advanced age, longer-term QOL and functional outcomes need to be evaluated. The ethical challenge is finding a delicate balance: on the one hand, avoiding ageism and providing a therapy to older patients that offers the only meaningful chance for improved survival, especially in early-stage disease, and on the other hand, avoiding overzealously providing a therapy with significant morbidity and mortality to older persons who are already at greater risk for functional loss and death.

ACKNOWLEDGMENTS

The author acknowledges the assistance of Jude K. A. des Bordes in the literature review relevant to this article.

REFERENCES

1. Gridelli C, Langer C, Maione P, et al. Lung cancer in the elderly. J Clin Oncol 2007;25(14):1898–907.
2. van Durme YM, Verhamme KM, Stijnen T, et al. Prevalence, incidence, and lifetime risk for the development of COPD in the elderly: the Rotterdam study. Chest 2009;135(2):368–77.
3. Dexter EU, Jahangir N, Kohman LJ. Resection for lung cancer in the elderly patient. Thorac Surg Clin 2004;14(2):163–71.
4. U.S. Census Bureau projected population of the United States by age and sex: 2000 to 2050. Available at: http://www.census.gov/population/www/projections/usinterimproj. Accessed February, 2009.
5. Rodin MB, Mohile SG. A practical approach to geriatric assessment in oncology. J Clin Oncol 2007;25(14):1936–44.

6. Extermann M, Hurria A. Comprehensive geriatric assessment for older patients with cancer. J Clin Oncol 2007;25(14):1824–31.
7. Association of Directors of Geriatric Academic Programs Status of Geriatrics Workforce Study. Available at: http://www.adgapstudy.uc.edu/Home.cfm. Accessed February, 2009.
8. SEER Stat Fact Sheets: lung and bronchus. Available at: http://seer.cancer.gov/statfacts/html/lungb.html. Accessed February, 2009.
9. Sugimura H, Yang P. Long-term survivorship in lung cancer: a review. Chest 2006;129(4):1088–97.
10. Chang MY, Mentzer SJ, Colson YL, et al. Factors predicting poor survival after resection of stage IA non-small cell lung cancer. J Thorac Cardiovasc Surg 2007;134(4):850–6.
11. SEER Fast Stats. Available at: http://seer.cancer.gov/faststats/selections.php. Accessed February, 2009.
12. Thomas P, Piraux M, Jacques LF, et al. Clinical patterns and trends of outcome of elderly patients with bronchogenic carcinoma. Eur J Cardiothorac Surg 1998;13(3):266–74.
13. Oliaro A, Leo F, Filosso PL, et al. Resection for bronchogenic carcinoma in the elderly. J Cardiovasc Surg (Torino) 1999;40(5):715–9.
14. Audisio RA, Zbar AP, Jaklitsch MT. Surgical management of oncogeriatric patients. J Clin Oncol 2007;25(14):1924–9.
15. Sullivan V, Tran T, Holmstrom A, et al. Advanced age does not exclude lobectomy for non-small cell lung carcinoma. Chest 2005;128(4):2671–6.
16. Suemitsu R, Takeo S, Hamatake M, et al. The perioperative complications for elderly patients with lung cancer associated with a pulmonary resection under general anesthesia. J Thorac Oncol 2009;4(2):193–7.
17. Cerfolio RJ, Bryant AS. Survival and outcomes of pulmonary resection for non-small cell lung cancer in the elderly: a nested case-control study. Ann Thorac Surg 2006;82(2):424–9 [discussion: 29–30].
18. Jaklitsch MT, Mery CM, Audisio RA. The use of surgery to treat lung cancer in elderly patients. Lancet Oncol 2003;4(8):463–71.
19. Limmer S, Hauenschild L, Eckmann C, et al. Thoracic surgery in the elderly—co-morbidity is the limit. Interact Cardiovasc Thorac Surg 2009;8(4):412–6.
20. Brunelli A, Socci L, Refai M, et al. Quality of life before and after major lung resection for lung cancer: a prospective follow-up analysis. Ann Thorac Surg 2007;84(2):410–6.
21. Sirbu H, Schreiner W, Dalichau H, et al. Surgery for non-small cell carcinoma in geriatric patients: 15-year experience. Asian Cardiovasc Thorac Ann 2005;13(4):330–6.
22. Hasse J, Wertzel H, Kassa M, et al. Thoracic cancer surgery in the elderly. Eur J Surg Oncol 1998;24(5):403–6.
23. Rostad H, Naalsund A, Strand TE, et al. Results of pulmonary resection for lung cancer in Norway, patients older than 70 years. Eur J Cardiothorac Surg 2005;27(2):325–8.
24. Jaklitsch MT, Pappas-Estocin A, Bueno R. Thoracoscopic surgery in elderly lung cancer patients. Crit Rev Oncol Hematol 2004;49(2):165–71.
25. Sawada S, Komori E, Nogami N, et al. Advanced age is not correlated with either short-term or long-term postoperative results in lung cancer patients in good clinical condition. Chest 2005;128(3):1557–63.
26. Kaplan RM, Ries AL, Reilly J, et al. Measurement of health-related quality of life in the national emphysema treatment trial. Chest 2004;126(3):781–9.
27. Myrdal G, Valtysdottir S, Lambe M, et al. Quality of life following lung cancer surgery. Thorax 2003;58(3):194–7.
28. Handy JR Jr, Asaph JW, Skokan L, et al. What happens to patients undergoing lung cancer surgery? Outcomes and quality of life before and after surgery. Chest 2002;122(1):21–30.
29. Aaronson NK, Ahmedzai S, Bergman B, et al. The European Organization for Research and Treatment of Cancer QLQ-C30: a quality-of-life instrument for use in international clinical trials in oncology. J Natl Cancer Inst 1993;85(5):365–76.
30. Bergman B, Aaronson NK, Ahmedzai S, et al. The EORTC QLQ-LC13: a modular supplement to the EORTC Core Quality of Life Questionnaire (QLQ-C30) for use in lung cancer clinical trials. EORTC Study Group on Quality of Life. Eur J Cancer 1994;30A(5):635–42.
31. Cella DF, Bonomi AE, Lloyd SR, et al. Reliability and validity of the functional assessment of cancer therapy-lung (FACT-L) quality of life instrument. Lung Cancer 1995;12(3):199–220.
32. Schipper H, Clinch J, McMurray A, et al. Measuring the quality of life of cancer patients: the Functional Living Index-Cancer: development and validation. J Clin Oncol 1984;2(5):472–83.
33. Hollen PJ, Gralla RJ, Kris MG, et al. Quality of life during clinical trials: conceptual model for the Lung Cancer Symptom Scale (LCSS). Support Care Cancer 1994;2(4):213–22.
34. Brazier JE, Harper R, Jones NM, et al. Validating the SF-36 health survey questionnaire: new outcome measure for primary care. BMJ 1992;305(6846):160–4.
35. Hays RD, Morales LS. The RAND-36 measure of health-related quality of life. Ann Med 2001;33(5):350–7.
36. Pollard WE, Bobbitt RA, Bergner M, et al. The sickness impact profile: reliability of a health status measure. Med Care 1976;14(2):146–55.
37. Sarna L, Cooley ME, Brown JK, et al. Symptom severity 1 to 4 months after thoracotomy for lung cancer. Am J Crit Care 2008;17(5):455–67, quiz 68.

38. Paull DE, Thomas ML, Meade GE, et al. Determinants of quality of life in patients following pulmonary resection for lung cancer. Am J Surg 2006;192(5):565–71.
39. Salati M, Brunelli A, Xiume F, et al. Quality of life in the elderly after major lung resection for lung cancer. Interact Cardiovasc Thorac Surg 2009;8(1):79–83.
40. Maione P, Perrone F, Gallo C, et al. Pretreatment quality of life and functional status assessment significantly predict survival of elderly patients with advanced non-small-cell lung cancer receiving chemotherapy: a prognostic analysis of the multicenter Italian lung cancer in the elderly study. J Clin Oncol 2005;23(28):6865–72.
41. Montazeri A, Milroy R, Hole D, et al. How quality of life data contribute to our understanding of cancer patients' experiences? A study of patients with lung cancer. Qual Life Res 2003;12(2):157–66.
42. Pirl WF, Temel JS, Billings A, et al. Depression after diagnosis of advanced non-small cell lung cancer and survival: a pilot study. Psychosomatics 2008; 49(3):218–24.
43. Gathinji M, McGirt MJ, Attenello FJ, et al. Association of preoperative depression and survival after resection of malignant brain astrocytoma. Surg Neurol 2009;71(3):299–303.
44. Pignay-Demaria V, Lesperance F, Demaria RG, et al. Depression and anxiety and outcomes of coronary artery bypass surgery. Ann Thorac Surg 2003; 75(1):314–21.
45. Goodwin JS, Zhang DD, Ostir GV. Effect of depression on diagnosis, treatment, and survival of older women with breast cancer. J Am Geriatr Soc 2004; 52(1):106–11.
46. Wedding U, Pientka L, Hoffken K. Quality-of-life in elderly patients with cancer: a short review. Eur J Cancer 2007;43(15):2203–10.
47. Wiener DC, Argote-Greene LM, Ramesh H, et al. Choices in the management of asymptomatic lung nodules in the elderly. Surg Oncol 2004;13(4):239–48.
48. Cykert S. Risk acceptance and risk aversion: patients' perspectives on lung surgery. Thorac Surg Clin 2004;14(3):287–93.
49. Schulte T, Schniewind B, Dohrmann P, et al. The extent of lung parenchyma resection significantly impacts long-term quality of life in patients with non-small cell lung cancer. Chest 2009;135(2): 322–9.
50. Leo F, Scanagatta P, Baglio P, et al. The risk of pneumonectomy over the age of 70. A case-control study. Eur J Cardiothorac Surg 2007;31(5):780–2.
51. Spaggiari L, Scanagatta P. Surgery of non-small cell lung cancer in the elderly. Curr Opin Oncol 2007; 19(2):84–91.
52. Jaklitsch MT, Bueno R, Swanson SJ, et al. New surgical options for elderly lung cancer patients. Chest 1999;116(Suppl 6):480S–5S.
53. Jaklitsch MT, DeCamp MM Jr, Liptay MJ, et al. Video-assisted thoracic surgery in the elderly. A review of 307 cases. Chest 1996;110(3):751–8.
54. Walter LC, Covinsky KE. Cancer screening in elderly patients: a framework for individualized decision making. JAMA 2001;285(21):2750–6.
55. Carey EC, Covinsky KE, Lui LY, et al. Prediction of mortality in community-living frail elderly people with long-term care needs. J Am Geriatr Soc 2008; 56(1):68–75.
56. Colice GL, Shafazand S, Griffin JP, et al. Physiologic evaluation of the patient with lung cancer being considered for resectional surgery: ACCP evidenced-based clinical practice guidelines (2nd edition). Chest 2007;132(Suppl 3):161S–77S.
57. Beshay M, Dorn P, Ris HB, et al. Influence of comorbidity on outcome after pulmonary resection in the elderly. Asian Cardiovasc Thorac Ann 2007;15(4): 297–302.
58. Cigolle CT, Langa KM, Kabeto MU, et al. Geriatric conditions and disability: the Health and Retirement Study. Ann Intern Med 2007;147(3):156–64.

Thoracic Surgery in the Elderly: Areas of Future Research and Studies

Joseph LoCicero III, MD[a,b,*], Jason Philip Shaw, MD[b]

KEYWORDS

• Elderly • Geriatrics • Thoracic surgery
• Clinical trials • Stress response

Geriatrics, first named and identified as a special field of knowledge in 1909, laid dormant through most of the twentieth century. A renaissance began in the mid-1970s, gaining strength over the next 3 decades. This renaissance was limited initially to the care of older patients within internal medicine, family medicine, psychiatry, and neurology. Only recently have surgeons realized that there is a separate and distinct need for a focus on geriatrics.

Much of the literature on surgical outcomes defines the elderly population as any adult aged more than 65 years. In the literature that deals with patient populations of octogenarians or nonagenarians, the data and conclusions often support the concept that a surgical team can perform operations on these groups with "acceptable results." These investigators feel that they are still fighting ageism among referring physicians and surgeons. They believe that the statement "we achieved acceptable results" should be sufficient to prove their hypothesis; however, some institutions that operate routinely on the oldest old are beginning to transcend ageism and are looking for ways not only to maintain "acceptable results" but also to optimize quality of life for the elderly.

The American Geriatrics Society (AGS), founded in 1942 specifically to advocate for better care for the elderly, defines the oldest old as persons aged 75 years and more. Individuals aged more than 75 years have less organ reserve and demonstrate a blunted response to stress. Nonetheless, age may not be as sensitive a predictor of adverse surgical outcomes as comorbidity, functional status, or other yet undetermined risk factors.

The concept of frailty emerged to describe a phenotype characterized by a vulnerability to acute stressors and an inability to mount an adequate compensatory physiologic response. Investigators describe a complex relationship among sarcopenia or age-related decline in lean muscle mass, physical activity, nutrition, and energy expenditure.[1] Although cardiopulmonary comorbidities may coexist in frail patients, frailty is a distinct entity with unique biologic underpinnings.[2] Many of the complex interactions such as immune responses, cellular mediators, and neuroendocrine processes that make frail patients vulnerable remain to be elucidated. Furthermore, it is hypothesized that frailty, if identified, may be reversible.

Frail elderly adults are at high risk for adverse events and functional deterioration following thoracic surgery for several reasons. Several physiologic factors contribute to the challenge of thoracic surgery in the elderly—the normal age-related decline in lung function, advanced chronic obstructive lung disease in lifelong smokers, and other comorbid diseases such as cardiac disease, diabetes, and osteoporosis. Thoracic surgery involves stress on multiple organ systems that often uncovers clinically unrecognized vulnerability to stress. Complications are most often respiratory or cardiac. Morbidity of the operation may lead to subsequent deterioration in global health and functional quality of life that extends beyond discharge from the hospital. Such morbidity and quality of life deterioration may

[a] SUNY Downstate, Brooklyn, NY, USA
[b] Maimonides Medical Center, 4802 Tenth Avenue, 4th Floor, Brooklyn, NY 11219, USA
* Corresponding author. Maimonides Medical Center, 4802 Tenth Avenue, 4th Floor, Brooklyn, NY 11219.
E-mail address: jlocicero@maimonidesmed.org (J. LoCicero III).

Thorac Surg Clin 19 (2009) 409–413
doi:10.1016/j.thorsurg.2009.07.003
1547-4127/09/$ – see front matter

result from the trauma of surgery, general anesthesia, or immobility during hospitalization rather than being the direct result of the pathology for which the procedure was indicated.

In addition, recovery from thoracic surgery requires muscle strength and physical activity to facilitate maneuvers such as deep breathing, coughing, and early ambulation to avoid the known complications of atelectasis, venous thrombosis, and pneumonia. Many frail elderly have gait disturbances, decreased lean body mass, and subtle neurocognitive deficits that make participation in postoperative rehabilitation difficult. An operation on such a vulnerable patient may incite a cascade of events that overwhelms the physiologic reserves and heralds a progression of functional and physiologic decline. If an elective surgical operation on an elderly patient is defined as a planned trauma, investigators may be able to examine problems of allostasis (the normal age-related decline in organ function) and homeostenosis (lack of the ability to mount a stress response) among frail elderly adults.

The AGS recognized the need for specialists to understand the special problems of the elderly. In the early 1990s, Dr. Dennis Jahnigen, Chief of Geriatrics at the University of Colorado School of Medicine and a widely respected leader in academic geriatrics, advanced the revolutionary idea that the next frontier for improving health care for older adults would lie not only in the subspecialties of internal medicine but also in surgery and certain related medical specialties.

Dr. Jahnigen sought to spark a similar change in other specialties that accounted for a large crucial segment of the care of older patients. Spurred by Dr. Jahnigen, the AGS and the John A. Hartford Foundation joined forces to create the project entitled Increasing Geriatrics Expertise in the Non-Primary Care Specialties, later changed to Increasing Geriatrics Expertise in Surgical and Related Medical Specialties and often shortened to simply the Geriatrics for Specialists project. The project began in 1992 with a planning grant. The Phase 1 grant ran from 1994 to 1997. It was renewed for Phase 2 from 1997 to 2001 and again for Phase 3 from 2001 to 2005. In Phase 3, the annual budget rose to almost $1.5 million, and several new programs were introduced. The project currently is in Phase 4 with an emphasis on expanding the research education of the practicing specialist.

The mission of the Hartford-funded Geriatrics for Specialists project is to improve the health care of elderly Americans by enhancing specialists' knowledge of geriatrics. Its specific objectives are to improve the amount and quality of geriatrics education received by residents in the surgical and related medical specialties, to identify and support specialty faculty in promoting geriatrics training and research within their own professional disciplines, and to assist certifying bodies and professional societies in improving the ability of their constituencies to care for elderly patients.

The Hartford-funded Geriatrics for Specialists project began to address the incredible need for quality specialty research by establishing the Research Agenda Setting Project (RASP). The RASP began in 2001 with selection of faculty members, one in each specialty, to serve as content experts. Their assignment was to review the present state of research on the geriatrics aspects of each specialty. A Senior Writing Group (SWG) consisting of one senior leader in each of the ten specialties was also appointed. The senior writer in each field was charged with assisting and guiding the content expert in conducting the literature review. The SWG also was responsible for identifying the cross-cutting issues and writing a first draft of that chapter.

The content experts met at the RAND Corporation in Santa Monica, California in February of 2001 to receive instruction in how to conduct a systematic literature review and how to classify research by type of study design. They developed preliminary search strategies, assisted by RAND librarians. During this process, many of the content experts, in consultation with the librarians, revised their search strategy and created new lists of titles, abstracts, and full articles. In a few instances, the content experts expanded their search independently. In all cases, reference lists from articles were searched for additional relevant earlier publications.

Content experts submitted drafts of literature reviews to the editors, who guided them in making revisions. These revised chapters formed the basis for a working conference in Potomac, Maryland in November 2001, which was cosponsored by the Agency for Health Care Research and Quality. The AGS invited five-person teams in each specialty to attend; each team was made up of the content expert, the senior writer, two at-large leaders in the specialty, and one geriatrician. Each content expert presented the major findings of the literature search. The specialty teams then met to critique the literature review and begin creating the research agenda. Preliminary research agendas were presented to the conference in plenary session. There were no face-to-face meetings after November of 2001. Considerable work and revision continued, supervised by the editors and the leadership of the Council of Surgical Specialties of the AGS. The first edition was published in 2004.[3] In that book, thoracic surgery was separated from cardiac surgery because of the dichotomous focus of the disciplines. Since then, project participants and leaders have updated the chapters, publishing a supplement in 2008.[4]

In the first edition of the RASP, multiple questions were posed for clinical researchers to consider when creating new studies. The main focus of these topics was to demonstrate the profound value of surgical procedures in the elderly population and to find ways to perform continuous process improvement that could be measured in a scientific manner. The chapter on general thoracic surgery first listed questions that are key to the expansion of knowledge in the surgical approach to the elderly patient (**Box 1**). The first two questions may be asked of any surgical discipline. The third question is directed at the thoracic surgical population but just as easily could be addressed to any discipline.

Specific research issues listed in **Box 2** include the development of assessment tools and preoperative preparation protocols to improve outcomes in the elderly to make surgical management of lung cancer in the oldest old acceptable from a risk standpoint. A complete list of the expanded research questions is provided in the Appendix to this article. Four levels of study magnitude and impact were identified. All of the proposed studies for general thoracic surgery fell into the highest two categories. D'Amico and LoCicero[5] summarized the research on thoracic surgery in the supplement to the RASP. They reiterated that little research has been done in a scientifically rigorous manner. What has been done barely begins to address any of the research questions.

To date, approaches to minimize risk or extend curative operations to the elderly have focused on making anesthesia or operative techniques safer or recognizing risk factors to exclude high-risk patients.

Box 1
Questions key to the expansion of knowledge in the surgical approach to the elderly patient

Basic key clinical research questions for any surgery in the elderly

How effective is preoperative preparation in improving the immediate surgical outcome for elderly patients?

What changes in perioperative care are needed to improve outcomes in the elderly surgical patient?

Basic key clinical research question for thoracic surgery in the elderly

To what extent do thoracic surgical operations improve quality of life outcomes in the elderly patient population?

Box 2
Research issues in surgical management of elderly patients

Development of an instrument to assess age-specific outcomes, functional status, and quality of life for elderly thoracic surgical patients

Incorporation of the age-specific instrument in ongoing surgical trials

Development and validation of a preoperative tool to assess the general function of the elderly patient having a major thoracic surgical procedure

Development and validation of preoperative optimization that addresses the most important risk factors for morbidity and mortality from thoracic surgical procedures

Randomized controlled trials in the elderly to evaluate minimally invasive techniques for pulmonary and esophageal operations

New surgical approaches to the management of thoracic disease, including minimally invasive surgical procedures (video-assisted thoracoscopic lobectomy) and limited resections (such as segmentectomy), have emerged largely in response to the need to minimize surgical risk and improve convalescence in elderly patients who might otherwise not be candidates for curative resection.[6] Efforts directed specifically at the frail elderly remain sparse. Currently, a survey of the Clinical Trials database[7] demonstrates how meager the research efforts are. Only one cardiac surgery and one general thoracic surgery trial is registered (**Box 3**).

Major research questions have been prepared for thoracic surgery. Only thoracic surgeons as research team leaders will be able to address these questions. It is incumbent on all thoracic surgeons to collaborate on providing solid data to the medical community so that elderly patients will benefit from their expertise.

APPENDIX

Research questions proposed in *New Frontiers in Geriatrics Research: An Agenda for Surgical and Related Medical Specialties* (2004) *and Supplement 1* (2008) are as follows:

Key Research Questions

How effective is preoperative preparation in improving the immediate surgical outcome for elderly patients?

What changes in perioperative care are needed to improve outcomes in the elderly thoracic surgical patient?

Box 3
Current registered cardiac and thoracic surgical trials specifically for elderly patients[a]

Thoracic Onco-Geriatric Assessment (TOGA) Trials

Institution(s): University of Wisconsin, Madison

Condition(s): Thoracic neoplasms (any)

Intervention: behavioral, Thoracic Onco-Geriatric Assessment (TOGA) tools

Description: to develop a reliable, physician and patient friendly, preoperative TOGA to predict surgical risk in geriatric oncology patients with thoracic neoplasms of the lung, esophagus, pleura, and thymus, modeled upon existing Comprehensive Geriatric Assessment (CGA) tools, including the Preoperative Assessment of Cancer in the Elderly (PACE)

ClinicalTrials.gov Identifier: NCT00591981

German Off Pump Coronary Artery Bypass in Elderly Study

Institution(s): German Off Pump Coronary Artery Bypass in Elderly Study Group, Institut für Klinisch-Kardiovaskuläre Forschung GmbH Deutsche Gesellschaft für Herz-, Thorax- und Gefäßchirurgie

Description: comparison of on-pump versus off-pump coronary revascularization for patients aged 75 years or older

Condition(s): heart disease

Intervention: other, coronary artery bypass grafting

ClinicalTrials.gov Identifier: NCT00719667

[a] Surveyed from http://ClinicalTrials.gov January 2, 2009.

To what extent do thoracic surgical operations improve quality of life outcomes in the elderly patient population?

Detailed Research Questions

Malignant diseases of the lungs

(Level A) (Level A is defined as important studies with hypothesis-testing intent using designs such as randomized controlled trials, certain non-randomized controlled trials, or cohort studies that focus on a single hypothesis.) Randomized controlled trials are needed of the effect on mortality and morbidity of the use of CT screening for elderly patients with high-risk factors for the development of cancer.

(Level B) (Level B is defined as important studies with hypothesis-generating intent using designs including exploratory, multi-targeted cohort and case-control studies; retrospective or prospective analysis of large databases; cross-sectional observational studies; time series; outcome studies; retrospective case series; or post hoc analyses of randomized controlled trials.) An instrument to assess age-specific outcomes, functional status, and quality of life for elderly patients who have lung cancer that is applicable to preoperative and postoperative situations needs to be developed and validated.

(Level A) Ongoing large therapeutic lung cancer trials need to incorporate the age-specific instrument described in ThoracicSurg 2.

(Level B) A preoperative tool to assess the general function of the elderly patient having a major pulmonary procedure needs to be developed and validated.

(Level B) A multivariate analysis using the Society of Thoracic Surgeons database or other collections of cases and aimed at defining the most important risk factors for adverse surgical outcomes should be performed. The instrument should include measures of the patient's functional capacity as well as pulmonary function.

(Level B) A method of preoperative optimization that addresses the most important risk factors for morbidity and mortality from pneumonectomy should be developed and tested.

(Level A) Randomized controlled trials are needed to compare the efficacy of preoperative optimization methods with current best medical practices. (Modification of this question in light of new research: This question should remain unmodified on the research agenda; however, over the previous 2 decades, a large amount of clinical experience has been gained regarding the use of induction therapy for non–small cell lung cancer. The following controversial issues should be addressed in clinical trials: the selection of patients for resection after induction therapy, the use of induction chemotherapy versus chemoradiotherapy, the use of induction chemotherapy for early stage disease, and the use of induction therapy as opposed to adjuvant therapy.)

(Level A) Randomized controlled trials are needed to evaluate video-assisted thoracic surgery techniques for lobectomy. The trials should compare outcomes, including long-term survival in elderly patients, with those of standard open procedures.

Benign diseases of the lungs

(Levels B, A) The effects of lung volume reduction procedures and their complications on elderly patients with chronic obstructive pulmonary disease need to be investigated in cohort studies that compare younger and older patients.

(Level A) Randomized trials are needed to evalate the efficacy of minimally invasive techniques nd compare them with standard thoracotomy for e management of empyema in elderly patients.

sophageal cancer

.evel B) Screening endoscopic trials should be erformed for elderly patients with longstanding eflux or a history of Barrett's esophagus to deterine whether early detection and treatment of igh-grade dysplasia is cost-effective.

(Levels B, A) Nonrandomized chemoprevention ials targeted specifically toward at-risk elderly atients should be continued, to be followed by randomized controlled trial of chemoprevention sing the most promising agent and comparing it ith usual care.

(Level B) The Society of Thoracic Surgeons atabase and other similar databases should be sed to gather data on the impact of age-related omorbidities and other factors related to operave management on the outcomes of esophagecomy for elderly patients.

(Level B) A national database for collecting orbidity and long-term survival rates of minimally vasive techniques for esophageal cancer should e established.

(Level B) Esophagectomy needs to be evaluated r effectiveness as a procedure for improving uality of life and preventing complications of aspition in elderly patients.

(Level B) Instruments to measure age-specific utcomes of surgery for esophageal cancer need be developed and validated. Functional status nd quality of life should be among the outcomes ssessed.

(Level A) Large clinical esophageal cancer trials hould incorporate the age-specific instruments escribed in ThoracicSurg 16.

(Level B) Esophagectomy could be used as model for highly complex surgical procedures the elderly patient to answer the following quesons: What makes the high-volume center able to rovide better care for elderly esophagectomy atients? Do high-volume centers achieve better urgical outcomes with the oldest old patients? what ways can care be improved for the elderly atient after esophagectomy? Once a formula for uccess is characterized, is it applicable to the are of elderly patients receiving other types of ajor operations?

enign esophageal disease

.evel B) A structured literature review should be erformed and a consensus conference between gastroenterologists and surgeons should be organized to establish criteria, based on symptoms and quality of life, for intervention in the management of gastroesophageal reflux disease, particularly in elderly patients.

(Level A) A prospective trial of laparoscopic antireflux surgery comparing elderly patients with younger matched control patients operated on during the same period should be performed to determine the suitability of this operation for the elderly patient.

Research in support of improved care (Level A) Genetic profiles should be collected on lung and esophageal cancer and paired with data on longterm survival to assess traditional staging and revise the staging system as needed.

(Level B) Observational studies are needed to compare new technologies for diagnosis and staging of lung and esophageal cancer with traditional methods.

REFERENCES

1. Fried LP, Tangen CM, Walston J, et al. Cardiovascular Health Study Collaborative Research Group. Frailty in older adults: evidence for a phenotype. J Gerontol A Biol Sci Med Sci 2001;56(3):M146–156.
2. Singh M, Alexander K, Roger VL, et al. Frailty and its potential relevance to cardiovascular care. Mayo Clin Proc 2008;83(10):1146–53.
3. Solomon DH, LoCicero J 3rd, Rosenthal RA, editors. New frontiers in geriatrics research: an agenda for surgical and related medical specialties. New York: American Geriatrics Society; 2004. Available at: http://www.americangeriatrics.org/specialists/NewFrontiers. Accessed September 10, 2009.
4. LoCicero J 3rd, Rosenthal RA, Katlic MR, editors. New frontiers in geriatrics research: an agenda for surgical and related medical specialties supplement 1. New York: American Geriatrics Society; 2008. Available at: http://www.americangeriatrics.org/specialists/NewFrontiers. Accessed September 10, 2009.
5. D'Amico TA, LoCicero J, 3rd. New frontiers in geriatrics research: an agenda for surgical and related medical specialties supplement 1. New York: Geriatrics Society; 2008. Available at: http://www.americangeriatrics.org/specialists/NewFrontiers. Accessed September 10, 2009.
6. Shaw JP, Dembitzer FR, Wisnivesky JP, et al. Video-assisted thoracoscopic lobectomy: state of the art and future directions. Ann Thorac Surg 2008;85(2):S705–709.
7. Available at: http://clinicaltrials.gov/ct2/search. Accessed September 10, 2009.

Index

Note: Page numbers of article titles are in **boldface** type.

Thorac Surg Clin 19 (2009) 415–418
doi:10.1016/S1547-4127(09)00064-4

Printed and bound by CPI Group (UK) Ltd, Croydon, CR0 4YY
03/10/2024
01040353-0014